AmiTREX — Pg 19

What Do You Do When the Medications Don't Work?

What Do You Do When the Medications Don't Work?

A Non-Drug Treatment of Dizziness,
Migraine Headaches, Fibromyalgia,
and Other Chronic Conditions

DR. MICHAEL L. JOHNSON

Board Certified Chiropractic Neurologist

JOKAMAR-JENAKE PUBLISHING
APPLETON

Medical disclaimer: The treatments and therapies described in this book are not intended to replace the services of a trained health professional. Your own physical condition and diagnosis may require specific modifications or precautions. Before undertaking any treatment or therapy, you should consult your physician or health care provider. Any application of the ideas, suggestions, and procedures set forth in this book are at the reader's discretion.

2nd edition June 2004

First published in the United States of America in 2003
by Jokamar-Jenake Publishing, Inc.

Library of Congress Cataloging-in-Publication Data
Johnson, Dr. Michael L.
What do you do when the medications don't work: a non-drug treatment of dizziness, migraine headaches, fibromyalgia, numbness, and other chronic conditions/Dr. Michael L. Johnson

Book design and edited by Joseph M. Johnson

Printed in the United States of America

In memory of my father-in-law,
JOSEPH M. CVENGROS (1929-1999)
Husband-Father-Educator

Table of Contents

1. **The Beginning**... 1
   Personal - Numbness- Growing up - Football-
   Sciatica - College - Pharmacy - Chiropractic - Palmer
2. **Onward and Upward**.. 9
   Appleton - Financing - Medical Doctors -
   HMO/PPO - Gonstead - Network -
   Dr. Carrick - Neurology - Green Bay -
   Manitowoc
3. **Right Brain/Left Brain**.................................... 19
   Left Brain - Broca's Speech Area -
   "Happy Brain" - Female/Male Brain -
   Right Brain - Frontal Lobe - Parietal
   Lobe - Plasticity - Cerebellum -
   Mesencephalon - Pons - Medulla
4. **Examination**...................................... 29
   Blood Pressure- SPO2 - Respiration - Pulse-
   Salivary pH - Chest Expansion - UA/Blood Work -
   Glucose - MSR - Vibration - Pinwheel - Muscle
   Strength - Weber - Rinne - Corneal Light Reflex -
   Pupillary Reflex - Accommodation - Pupil Size -
   Rapid Eye Movement - Cover/Uncover - Occular
   motion - Peripheral vision - V/A Ratio - OPK -
   Blind Spot - Olfactory perception - Facial -
   Hypoglossal - Romberg's Sign - Arm Slap - Past
   Pointing - Piano - Supination/Pronation - Heel
   tap - Heel to Toe Walk - Heel Down Shin -
   Temporal Lobe - Parietal Lobe - Abdominal -
   Bruits - Orthopedic Exams

5. **Treatment Modalities**............................... 47
   Unilateral Manipulation - Auditory
   Stimulation - Visual Stimulation - T.E.N.S.
   Heat - Ultrasound - IST - Warm/Cold
   Calorics - UBE - Olactory Stimulation -
   Visual Imagery - Mirror Imagery - Spin
   Therapy - Oxygen - Ultimate Eye Filters
6. **Vertigo/Dizziness**.................................... 57
   Vertigo Statistics - Canalith Training -
   Receptors - CIS - Caloric - Visual Imagery -
   George - Rita - Barb - Char - Esther
7. **Migraine Headaches**................................. 69
   Classical - Common - CSD - Cause - Jesse -
   Alice - Ginny - Jean - Sandy - Susan -
   Christopher
8. **Fibromyalgia**.. 83
   Fibromyalgia - Mesencephalon - Sleep -
   Light Sensitivity - Darlene - Christie -
   Linda - Diane - Paula Jean - Lana -
   Janie - Laura
9. **Other Chronic Cases**................................ 111
   Treatments - Straight/Mixer - Marlene -
   Lawrence - Corrine - Maxine
10. **Chiropractic and Strokes**........................ 121
    Neurology - The Post - Number of Strokes -
    Number of Deaths - NCMIC - WCA

11. **Nutrition**... 127
     Calcium - EFA - Magnesium - Selenium -
     Zinc - Vitamin A - Vitamin B1 - B2 -
     B6 - B12 - Vitamin C - D - E - K - Biotin -
     Chroline - Chromium - Copper - Folic
     Acid - Inositol - Iodine - Iron -Manganese-
     Niacin - PABA - Pantothenic Acid -
     Phosphorus - Potassium - Caffeine -
     Sugar/Aspartame - Protein - Alcohol -
     Detoxification - Elimination Diet/Food
     Allergies - Water
12. **Prayer**.. 145

Chapter 1:
The Beginning

"God heals, and the doctor takes the fee."
-Benjamin Franklin

What do you do when the medications don't work? What do you do when the medical doctor tells you that he has prescribed every medication possible and not one of them has provided relief? What do you do when the medical doctor tells you that "it's all in your head," meaning that it's a psychosomatic illness, or that "it's arthritis and you'll have to learn live with it?" What do you do? I'll tell you what you do: you suffer. How do I know? I have suffered.

Early in 1989, I developed severe migraine headaches while eating lunch at a restaurant near my office. All of a sudden, I began to feel a visual change in my eye. My best description of this change would be the appearance of "squiggly lines." After about twenty minutes, I lost the vision in my left eye. I ran into the bathroom suffering an intense pain. It was as if someone was pounding a spike into my left eye. I started to vomit profusely. When I say vomit, I mean projectile vomiting - all over the walls, all over the sink, all over everything. Following the restaurant ordeal, I would experience a migraine headache once or twice weekly. As time progressed, I noticed that the headaches were increasing in intensity and frequency. I tried treatment after treatment: numerous medications, vitamins, herbs, and various chiropractic techniques but nothing provided even the slightest form of relief. It felt as though my migraines were becoming worse with each new treatment that I tried. I would go on trips with my family and have to sit in a dark room while they were having a good time. After two years of continually worsened headaches, I decided to search for a chiropractic technique that would help my condition. Perhaps by first helping myself, I could then help my patients who suffered from migraine headaches.

I attended a seminar in which the speaker stated that in order to become a great chiropractor, I would have to master every technique in chiropractic. At that time, there were approximately thirty techniques. I went on a quest to find the best technique, perhaps a technique that would combine them all, in an effort to relieve my suffering. During the entire spring and summer of 1990, I attended a seminar every weekend. By that time, my wife and I had three children, and naturally, my wife was not happy. Before I continue, let me start at the beginning.

I grew up in a small town in Upper Michigan. As is the case in many small towns, when you become a freshman in high school, the football coach does not ask you to play football - he tells you. Small towns have small schools, and small schools cannot afford to have a freshman team and junior varsity team. Freshman and sophomores formed what we called the "hamburger squad," "hamburger" in this case meaning raw meat. The members of the hamburger squad got the crap beat out of them every day in practice, allow-ing them the privilege of standing on the sidelines to watch the game every Friday or Saturday night. Football practice would begin in August with two-a-day practices until the first game. Beginning in August of my sophomore year, a sharp pain shot down my right arm whenever I tackled another player. This is normally called a "stinger" in football circles. As the season progressed, my stingers worsened. They eventually became so severe that my hand would be numb for two or three days at a time.

I would call in sick to school so I would not have to go to foot-ball practice. After two or three weeks of not making it to Tuesday or Wednesday football practice, the coach was not happy. I barely made it through my sophomore year. I survived, but the numbness would come and go for a few weeks after the football season had ended.

In my junior year, the numbness and paresthesia returned dur-ing the second week of football practice. This time, the numbness would last for a week. I would lose all of the feeling in my hand. I was the tight end on the football team and I would often be wide open for a pass, but having no feeling in my right hand, I would drop the ball. The paresthesia in my right hand and arm lasted well into basketball season. Following my junior year of basketball sea-son, I decided not to play football my senior year. After playing three years of football - granted, not very good football - I was ostracized for not going out for "the team". I was ostracized not only by other football players and coaches but also by many adults in the community.

The summer of my senior year, I developed lower back pain radiating down into my right leg. By the time basketball season began, the lower back pain and sciatica were quite severe, and I decided to see our family doctor. Our medical doctor was not the most personable man in the world. A patient would go into his office, wait approximately thirty minutes, and then be shuttled into another room. After another fifteen to twenty minutes, the doctor would enter with note cards, ask about the symptom, write on the note cards, and then prescribe some sort of medication. When I went to see him for my lower back pain, he had mentioned something along the lines of surgery. Even as a 17 year-old high school senior, something about surgery just didn't feel right to me. I talked it over with my mom and stepfather, and my stepfather recommended that I see his chiropractor. My stepfather had played football in high school, and as a result, he suffered from chronic neck pain. I had never been to a chiropractor before, nor did I have any clue what a chiropractor did, but anything was better than surgery.

I went to see Dr. Fred Schwartz in Ironwood, Michigan. He took my history, performed an examination, and x-rayed my lower back. He told me that I had a "pinched nerve" and proceeded to treat me by utilizing ultrasound and spinal manipulation. After five or six visits, I felt great! I no longer had lower back pain or leg pain. Life went on.

I graduated from high school in 1977 and decided to become a pharmacist. My maternal grandfather had owned a pharmacy in Bayfield, Wisconsin from 1930 until 1952. I believe that when one pursues a field or profession, one should strive to be the very best. I felt the best pharmacy school in Michigan at that time was Ferris State College in Big Rapids, Michigan. Sight unseen, I would attend Ferris. I never bothered to look at any other schools. All of my friends decided to attend college at Michigan Tech in Houghton, MI or Northern Michigan University in Marquette, MI, which were only a few hours from home. Ferris, located ten hours away in downstate Michigan, seemed light-years away from my hometown.

During my freshman year in college, my participation in gym class began to aggravate my lower back pain and sciatica. I went to the health center at the college and explained my condition, and the doctor prescribed pain medication. I was handed a note exempting me from class and given a board to put under my bed. I was also told that I would need a release from my medical doctor stating that I suffered from lower back pain. I asked if I could just get the release from my chiropractor, but the doctor at the health center insisted that the release be obtained directly from my medical doctor, NOT the chiropractor. I went home and told the medical doctor about the condition, and he wrote a prescription and the release statement. Once again, my medical doctor talked about the possibility of surgery if things did not go well. I was afraid to tell him about the great results that I had with Dr. Schwartz.

During my second term at Ferris, I had a gut feeling that I did not want to be a pharmacist. Having many friends and patients as pharmacists, I know that it is an excellent field, but my goal from a young age was to own a business. This entrepreneurial spirit was in my blood: my dad owned a small GM dealership and my grandfather had owned a Ford dealership. Besides, I'm better at giving orders than taking them. As I became familiar with the pharmaceutical field, I found that the chances of achieving my goal in pharmacy were slim. At that time, large corporations with pharmacies, like K-Mart, Walgreens, and Shopko, were quickly spreading throughout the Midwest. I could only envision myself working for some big company, counting pills into a bottle, and collecting a paycheck. Many years later, in the Sunday, February 9, 2003 edition of the *Green Bay Press Gazette*, there was an article entitled, "Druggist Struggle for Career Happiness." The article went on to state that "retail pharmacists may be highly paid and are hot with recruiters, but many are having difficulties finding happiness on the job."

Although I decided not to become a pharmacist, I was certain that I wanted a career in the healthcare field. I looked into physical therapy, but I could not see myself working in a hospital. For some time I seriously considered becoming a medical doctor, but I remembered the poor bedside manner of my childhood doctor. He always seemed to prescribe the same blue and yellow pills. As I was beginning to think I had exhausted all of my options, my friend started telling me about his brother, a chiropractor in Lower Michigan. With his information and the good experience I had with Dr. Schwartz, I decided to become a chiropractor. I set out to find the best chiropractic college in the country.

After speaking to many chiropractors and writing to many chiropractic colleges, I decided to attend the Palmer College of Chiropractic in Davenport, IA. About the same time I decided to be a chiropractor, *60 Minutes* did a very negative report on chiropractic. One of my roommates and I were watching it when he asked, "Are you still going to be a chiropractor after watching this?" I told him that this had not been my experience and I would decide for myself.

I considered returning to Ferris State to finish my undergrad studies and receive my Bachelor of Science degree, but when I looked at my course curriculum for my final year, it seemed to include many "non-essential studies." I also could not afford to stay at Ferris another year. At the time I applied to Palmer College of Chiropractic, an undergraduate only needed to have completed two years of pre-chiropractic studies to be accepted. I applied to Palmer during my junior year, and I was then accepted in the spring of 1980. Looking back, I regret leaving my friends at Ferris, but I am one to make a decision and move forward. In February of 1980, I left Ferris State College, took a month off, and enrolled at Palmer College of Chiropractic on April 4, 1980. During my first few weeks at Palmer, I met some wonderful people. Palmer's climate was much different from many other colleges in that the majority of students would not take the summers off. They would complete the four years of material in three years, so it was similar to a high school class. You would be with the same 150 classmates throughout your studies. You could take a quarter off and drop back to the next class, or you could take as many quarters off as you liked and re-enter. While I was attending Palmer, I decided to join the Gonstead Club. Gonstead is one of the thirty techniques in chiropractic. I decided on Gonstead because it gave me an opportunity to work with doctors in the field. My goal was to be the best.

In my sixth quarter at Palmer, after dating Michele since my senior year in high school, my wife and I were married. She had just graduated from college and was looking for a teaching position in Davenport, IA. All she could find was a parochial school position at a salary of $6000 per year. Michele taught first grade during the day and worked as a waitress at night while I worked at a trucking firm loading semi-trailers. Needless to say, we did not have a lot of money to get through school. I graduated from Palmer in March of 1983. While I was waiting for Michele to finish teaching, I worked for a chiropractor named Dr. Herb Wood in Davenport. This was a very positive experience because I could observe a doctor in practice. Though we had never been there before, Michele and I decided to move to Appleton, WI to start a practice. I don't know if you have ever had a gut instinct, but this decision was one of those gut feelings for us.

Chapter 2:
Onward and Upward

"I feel no care of coin;
Well doing is my wealth;
My mind to me an empire is,
While grace affordeth health."
-Robert Southwell: *Content and Rich*

We moved to Appleton on June 15, 1983, in the middle of the hottest summer on record. We found a brand new duplex to rent with no air conditioning. I made up a beautiful business plan and went from bank to bank looking for a $25,000 loan to open my practice. I found a great location that I wanted to rent, but the space really was not for rent – the vacant area was upstairs. The tenant in the building didn't need the ground level area that I was interested in, and he was willing to let me lease it. Ironically, two pharmacists owned the building. Mylan Sinclair and Morris Gabbert owned Appleton Pharmacy, an Appleton institution since the 1950s. Looking back, I could not have asked for better landlords.

Now, my only problem was obtaining the finances. Being young and inexperienced, I walked into the first few banks with my loan portfolio, expecting to receive a resounding "yes" and be on my way. After visiting the tenth bank and receiving my tenth resounding "NO," I started to become a little discouraged. On top of that, when I came back to the hotel, I noticed that the back of my suit collar was sticking straight up and no one had bothered to let me know. I imagined the loan officers' thoughts: "Here's a twenty-four year-old, flunky kid just out of school, coming in to a bank and expecting a $25,000 loan, yet he doesn't even know how to wear a suit!" I didn't think we would be able to make it, but my wife called her father and my father-in-law promised $10,000 in collateral. My dad contributed another $5,000. We got the note, signed a lease, and on September 1, 1983, I opened my practice.

I had a friend, a chiropractor in Manitowoc, Wisconsin, who also utilized the Gonstead Technique. He had opened his clinic a year earlier, so he taught me how to get my name out to the public. I started advertising in the newspaper, hired a consulting firm, and joined various organizations. In my first week of practice, the Valley Nurse's Association filed a complaint with the state board about my advertising. My ads simply explained symptoms, such as sciatica, lower back pain, and headaches, and they described how a chiropractor could treat each condition. They were very general and **very** non-threatening, but they were apparently threatening enough to the Nurse's Association. I received a letter of investigation and dismissal about a month later. Many years later, I found that another chiropractor, whose wife belonged to the Valley Nurse's Association, was actually behind the complaint.

Along with my advertising and networking, I hooked up with a local high school football team as the team doctor, and the practice grew. After about six months, we were rocking: the office was treating about 200 patients per week. I decided to call a few local M.D.'s and ask them to lunch to discuss mutual patients and how I would be able to help them with chiropractic care. I learned in 1983 that medical doctors did not like chiropractors; in fact, they hated chiropractors. Most of the medical doctors that I called simply refused to speak to me. A few barked at me, and a couple swore at me. So much for professional courtesy - apparently they were absent from class the day it was taught in medical school.

In the past twenty years, I have learned that some medical doctors have excellent bedside manner and some are pompous jerks. Patients have told me that many medical doctors have very condescending attitudes – some doctors even swear at patients. Patients have also said that their medical doctors do not want to be asked **any** questions because the doctor feels that the patient is undermining his or her authority. I recently had an 86 year-old woman who had been treated by many medical doctors present to my office. She had nothing positive to report about medical doctors - only that they were extremely rude. Unfortunately, I hear this all too often. My advice is to follow the "golden rule" - treat people the way you would like to be treated.

When I became a chiropractic neurologist, I sent out information to medical doctors on the neurology courses I had taken. In return, I received a letter from a local orthopedic surgeon accusing me of being a "medical scam artist." What he did not realize was that I had successfully treated many of his post-surgical patients whom he did not help. Many of his former patients had actually gotten worse following his "surgical intervention."

Many women suffering with fibromyalgia and chronic fatigue syndromes said that their medical doctors told them that their symptoms were "all in their head." If they would just "get out and exercise," they wouldn't have these symptoms. Many have been told that they have a "psychosomatic illness" or that they were simply "looking for attention." When I examined these women, they all had severe neurological signs and many positive neurological tests. Just because the doctor's medical knowledge is limited to the point that he or she cannot or will not determine positive findings, does not mean the patient is "faking it" or is a "malingerer." In many cases, patients like these will present to a medical doctor who won't even perform an exam, take x-rays, or perform any type of lab tests. Are all medical doctors like this? No, as I have mentioned earlier, some medical doctors are excellent. Someone needs to inform the rest to get off their pedestals and listen to their patients.

Medicine is unparalleled when it comes to acute care (accidents, heart attacks, stroke, etc.), but drops the ball in treating chronic conditions.

Things were up and running in Appleton. I had been in practice for about four years, but some of my patients were not getting any better. A few patients were even getting worse, and this **really** bothered me. By 1987, I had my fill with the Gonstead technique, and I began to search for a different chiropractic technique that would better help my patients. At the same time, the State of Wisconsin passed a law mandating chiropractic care into all health insurance companies, including HMOs. A guy that I played basketball with at the YMCA was working with one of the HMOs, and he asked me to join. I was reluctant and decided to sit it out and let the dust settle. If things looked good down the road, I would join, but at that time, it was too much, too fast. Unfortunately, this decision was one of the biggest mistakes of my life. I didn't see the future coming, and it smacked me right upside the head. (Currently, HMO/PPOs cover 80% of the population in Northeastern Wisconsin. It's very difficult to help patients when your name is not on their list of doctors.)

In the spring of 1988, I realized that I had made a mistake, and I asked this gentleman if I could be a part of the HMO. Unfortunately, he turned me down flat. For the next fifteen years I would continually ask to be included as a participating provider, only to be turned down repeatedly, even after becoming a board-certified chiropractic neurologist. I met with him in March of 2002 to ask to be included one last time, and his response was: "How do I know if you're better than any other chiropractor that we have in our plan?" Hmm…let me see…probably because I have over 750 hours in neurological studies and 3500 hours in postgraduate education, I'm a board-certified chiropractic neurologist after completing a grueling twelve-hour written essay AND a one-hour oral practical, plus I'm getting many of the chronic pain patients in your HMO/PPO better when no other doctor is able to.

After five years of practicing the Gonstead Technique, I felt I had finally found a chiropractic technique that would improve my success rate. It was called ASBE (Applied Spinal Biomechanical Engineering). The name sure sounded impressive. I became a member of the American Academy of Applied Spinal Biomechanical Engineering, or A.A.A.S.B.E., for short. Using the ASBE technique, I would take twelve to sixteen x-rays of one patient. The instructor who developed this technique seemed to justify the amount of x-rays by stating that a doctor needs to see all aspects of a patient's spinal biomechanics. Because of the new technique, I purchased a new x-ray machine that emitted much less radiation. I attended special seminars sponsored by Kodak to learn to reduce radiation as much as possible, and away I went into the "I can now heal the world" sunset.

It was about this time that I developed severe migraine headaches. As time progressed, I had noticed that the headaches were becoming more intense and more frequent. Although I was performing my ASBE exercises and was being treated by a local chiropractor, my migraine headaches continually worsened. ASBE didn't seem to be working, and I decided to search for the "best technique" in chiropractic for the last time.

In September of 1990, I attended a seminar on Network Chiropractic. Network Chiropractic was a low-force technique that used a number of phases administered by the practicing doctor. A structural adjustment, which is what most people think of chiropractic (popping and cracking), may or may not follow. The added bonus to Network Chiropractic was that it relieved my migraine headaches somewhat, and I was very excited to help others with similar conditions. The problem with Network Chiropractic was that it was considered very "new age," and in the conservative, Republican region of Northeast Wisconsin, it did not go over well. As a joke, I made a video in which patients seem to be flipping around on a chiropractic table, but this was one of the most foolish things I have ever done. The state association obtained the video and turned it over to the Examining Board, which began to hold hearings on Network Chiropractic. The first hearing was held in December of 1992, but it did not get much press, so they held another hearing in March of 1993. The Wisconsin Chiropractic Association certainly got their publicity at that hearing, as my face was plastered all over the local newspapers the next day. In addition, things were not going well in my office. Patients were not accepting this "new age" technique, although it had provided me with some relief from my migraine headaches, and my negative press was no help. The media needs two things to sell papers: a "good guy" and a "bad guy." God help you if you're ever the "bad guy."

During the hearings in March of 1993, Ted Robinson, lead attorney for Network Chiropractic, came up to me and told me that Network Chiropractic was going to "disassociate" itself from me. In other words, I was going to be the fall guy. That was the end of my association with Network Chiropractic. I felt that I was being hung out to dry, even though everything I did was done at the Network Chiropractic seminars. The board and the state association attempted to ban Network Chiropractic from the state of Wisconsin, but they failed to do so. Along with three other Network chiropractors in Wisconsin, I sued the Wisconsin Chiropractic Association and its executive director Russ Leonard, and we settled out of court. In Leonard's mind, we may have won the battle, but he was going to win the war. To this day, Russ Leonard has nothing positive to say about me. Whenever patients call and ask about me, he scares them away. Years ago, I tried to rejoin the Wisconsin Chiropractic Association to move beyond our past differences. Leonard, however, would have nothing to do with it.

After Network, I found a doctor in the area who was treating approximately 1500 patients per week. He wouldn't tell me what he was doing, but I heard that he was using telemarketing in his practice. His office would call a random number from the telephone book, introduce his clinic, and offer the person a free spinal screening. In December of 1993, I began using telemarketing to attract new patients to my practice. Telemarketing saved my practice in the early 90s, as the power of the HMOs was increasing every year.

I again began to search for the perfect technique to relieve my migraine headaches and serve my patients at a higher level. In 1996, I decided to incorporate a medical doctor into my practice. I started one of the first clinics in the country to have a chiropractor, a medical doctor, and a physical therapist under one roof. Friends of mine who were medical doctors and chiropractors said it would **never** work. It did, and I have never looked back.

The first medical doctor hired was an "old school" doctor who lasted about a week. I could tell he was uneasy working with a chiropractor. The second doctor that was hired was a board-certified psychiatrist. I got along with him very well and we worked together on a number of cases.

In one particular case, we were able to diagnose a patient with Arnold-Chiari syndrome. Arnold-Chiari syndrome occurs when the cerebellum infiltrates down through the hole in the skull, called the foramen magnum. This patient presented for care complaining of cervical spine pain radiating down into the arm. He would get better, then worse, and then better again. After six or eight weeks, I referred him to our medical doctor, which is the standard procedure if conservative care is not working. Our medical doctor ordered an MRI of the cervical spine that revealed nothing, but when he ordered the MRI of the head, cervical syndrome was discovered. We immediately referred him to a neurosurgeon.

Our current medical doctor is a bariatric specialist (a physician who specializes in obesity), and she is a gem! She is easy to work with, she is very thorough, and the patients love her. Many patients who have been struggling with weight loss for years lose 40-90 pounds following her treatment, and they keep the weight off afterwards. If you would like more information on bariatric physicians, visit the American Society of Bariatric Physicians website at www.asbp.org.

In November of 1997, I hired an associate who told me about Dr. Ted Carrick, the country's leading chiropractic neurologist and chiropractic's only neurological fellow. Typically, a chiropractic neurologist serves in the same consulting manner as a medical neurologist. The difference is that the therapies or applications of a chiropractic neurologist do not include drugs or surgery. As a result, certain conditions are more customarily seen by a chiropractic neurologist as opposed to medical neurologist and vice versa.

My associate had been taking a number of neurology courses taught by Dr. Carrick, and he asked me if I would be interested in attending with him. I explained that I had already taken numerous neurology courses in the past fourteen years, all of which taught one thing: a chiropractor should assess the patient and refer them to a medical neurologist. I informed him that I didn't need a 300-hour course to teach me something that I already knew how to do. He insisted that Dr. Carrick's course was different. "Well, I have tried everything else, so I might as well take a look at this," I said. I was confident that this seminar would be no different from the others, but I accompanied my associate to satisfy him. We arrived at the seminar and sat with about 500 other doctors in a college gymnasium. Dr. Carrick proceeded to talk about neuron theory, which I had never heard of previously. Having not even heard of these conditions and neurological facts in my four years at Palmer College, I became frustrated and angry. As a doctor, I thought I should know **all** of this material, especially as a chiropractor who supposedly specializes in the nervous system. What really put me over the top is when Dr. Carrick administered "grand rounds" in which he would examine and treat patients.

The first patient he treated that morning was a 79 year-old male who had suffered a stroke that paralyzed the left side of his body. Because of the stroke, the only word that this man could speak was "ninety-nine." Dr. Carrick held up a pencil and asked the man what it was, and the man's response was "ninety-nine." "Ninety-nine" was his response to every question. After examining the man, Dr. Carrick explained how he would treat this stroke patient. At the next seminar, the man returned and was 90% improved. He could speak in clear sentences and knew what a pencil was. Witnessing Dr. Carrick's treatment proved to me the effectiveness of this method. My belief in neurology was further solidified when after I was treated, my migraine headaches disappeared. After nine years of suffering migraine headaches 2-3 times per week, many times to the point of extreme nausea, I am happy to report that I have not suffered a migraine headache since 1998.

I elected to attend seminars with Dr. Carrick in Dallas once a month for the next three years. I was so committed to using neurology in my practice that I had all of my associate doctors attend with me. After two or three months of seminars, I came back to Appleton fired up, thinking I could cure the world. Little did I know that I was only beginning my journey. I placed advertisements in the newspaper, one or two of my migraine patients really responded to care. I started to get cocky, thinking that I had the answer to migraine headaches. I ran a testimonial ad in the newspaper and received a response from a 21 year-old female with severe migraine headaches. Upon examination, I observed that she had a severe left exophoria. When you move a pencil toward a patient's eyes, the eyes should follow the pencil to the midline and hold there. A left exophoria occurs when the left eye moves to the midline, then bounces out. I was rather new to neurology, and I thought that the right brain controls the left eye. I reasoned that since the right brain controls the left eye, the cause of my patient's migraine headaches must be a decrease in the firing, or impulses, in the right brain. I chose to adjust this patient on the left side to excite the left cerebellum, which in turn will excite the right brain.

Let me tell you, this is **not** how you treat a migraine headache patient. The next visit, the patient came back and could not open her jaw. In addition, her headaches were worse. This patient never returned, and I cannot blame her. I was too ignorant to realize that I was only scratching the surface of neurology. I needed to dig deeper before I truly could treat patients with migraine headaches. Now that I know what to do with this type of patient, I would love to have another chance, but I guess it was all part of the learning experience.

Because things were going so well, I opened an office in Green Bay, WI in February of 1998. In May of 1999, I opened a third office in Manitowoc, WI. I had a number of chiropractic associates at that time, along with a physical therapist and a medical doctor. The service that a physical therapist provides is very beneficial to the patient, but physical therapy and chiropractic neurology don't mix. A chiropractic neurologist usually will treat one side of the body to increase impulses to the same-side of the cerebellum and opposite side of the brain. A physical therapist, however, is taught to treat the area of pain. I have had many cases in which a patient had right shoulder pain and the physical therapist was treating the right shoulder. The true problem was a decrease in the frequency of firing, or impulses, in the left cerebellum and right-brain. Therefore, one would want to treat the left side of the body, not the right. The physical therapist would actually increase the firing of the right cerebellum and left-brain by treating the right shoulder region. The right side of the body is controlled by the left brain. If a person is experiencing or perceiving pain on the right side of the body, it means that the left-brain is firing at a very high rate. You would want to increase the frequency of firing of the opposite (right) brain, so you would adjust or treat the patient on the left side and the left side only. Treating the right side usually will make the patient worse.

Chapter 3:
Right Brain/Left Brain

"I have good health, good thoughts, and good humour, thanks be to God Almighty."
-William Byrd: *Diary*

The right-brain controls the left side of the body, and the left-brain controls the right side of the body. The right-brain is the creative and emotional hemisphere, and the left-brain is the analytical and judgmental hemisphere. The right-brain works with information that is new to an individual, and the left-brain works with familiar information.

The left-brain controls our language information, including the

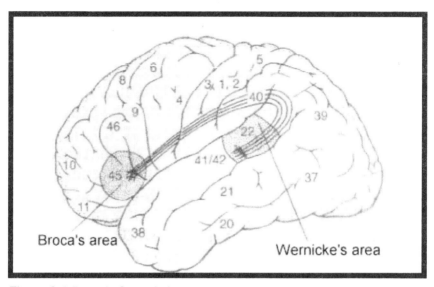

Figure 3-1 Broca's Speech Area

ability to read and speak. Broca's speech area, the area that allows you to communicate, is located in the left frontal lobe (area 45) of the brain (figure 3-1). When fibromyalgia and other chronic pain patients present to my office, I ask them if they have trouble expressing what they would like to say. Whenever I find a left-brain deficit, they will always answer "yes," wondering how I would know this. I explain to them that Broca's speech area is located in the left temporal lobe, and this area allows you to communicate. When someone can visualize a word but cannot get it out of his mouth, Broca's speech area is not firing the way that it should. This means that there is a lack of impulses in that particular region of the brain. The person does not have a brain tumor, which is a hard lesion, but they have a soft lesion. A soft lesion is a lack of firing, or impulses, in a particular section of the brain. Wernicke's area of the brain (area 22) allows you to comprehend what is being said to you. The arcuate faciculus connects Broca's area to Wernicke's area.

The left-brain controls math skills and processes information

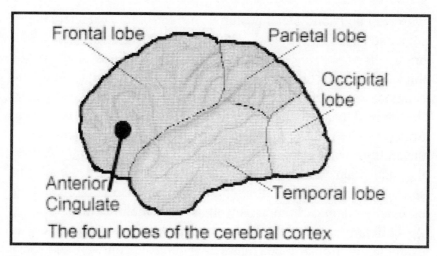

The four lobes of the cerebral cortex

Figure 3-2

from detailed facts. The fact that you enjoy your surroundings is dominant left-brain. The left-brain is not interested in trivial activities or environments, but it is very happy in a comfort zone and loves repetition and systems. Computers are a good fit with the left-brain. I have not met a person who works with computers and is not left-brain dominant. The left-brain is your "happy brain," and if it is not firing at a high rate, you will probably be depressed. In many cases, people who are left brain dominant (left brain over-firing) are not animated in their speech patterns. Their voice will sound very dull and monotone.

The female brain is more developed on the left side, and female brains are much more developed than male brains in general. I am not joking - this is a neurological fact. Besides, haven't you ever heard of women's intuition? Females have a much more developed anterior cingulate. (figure 3-2) The anterior cingulate allows for caring and compassion. Understand what I mean? Overall, females are definitely more caring and compassionate than males. Males have a much more developed angular gyrus which allows them a greater mechanical aptitude.

The right-brain controls non-verbal communication. The ability to read body and facial posture is a right-brain characteristic. If someone says "I love you" with a mean, nasty snarl, your right-brain tells you, "Hey, maybe they don't love you as much as you think." The right brain controls social behavior; it tells you if your behavior is appropriate for the environment that you are in. Withdrawal behavior, also known as negative behavior, is controlled by the right-brain. Drawing and reading comprehension - the ability to understand the meaning of a story - are controlled by the right-brain. The right-brain processes very complex math reasoning, as in abstract math. The right-brain also controls humor, especially complex humor, as well as gross motor skills.

Different areas of the brain also have specific functions. For example, the frontal lobe (figure 3-3) controls your self and social ego and determines your personality. The frontal lobe also initiates

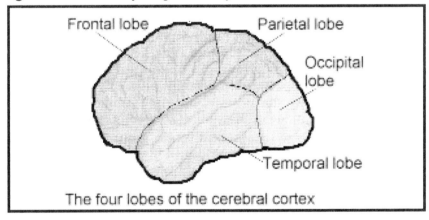

The four lobes of the cerebral cortex

Figure 3-3

feelings of strain and strength.

Physical, emotional, and chemical stress adversely affect the brain by causing a decrease in the frequency of firing, or impulses. When someone is under emotional stress, the adrenal medulla releases cortisol, a substance that is toxic to the hippocampus. The hippocampus is located deep within the temporal lobe, the part of the brain that controls memory. This is why people have trouble with their memory when they are under severe stress.

The temporal lobe also controls speech, verbal comprehension, and acoustic attentiveness, or understanding of noise and music. It deals with short and long-term memory. Long-term memory is located in the lower or inferior aspect of the temporal lobe, while short-term memory is located in the upper or superior aspect. The temporal lobe is also active with vision.

The parietal lobe processes sensory input from the environment. Another part of the brain, the occipital lobe, is located in the back part of the brain and receives input regarding vision.

In the January 2002 *Newsweek* article titled "Rewiring Your Gray Matter," author Shirley Begley states that you can "teach an old brain new tricks."

"It is the dawning realization that a brain older than three years is not a rigid structure that scientists long thought, but a malleable plastic organ. Ever since the 1950s, one of the great themes of neuroscience has been that neurons of the cortex matured during the critical period and the first few years of life, and that the brain's organization did not change after that," says neurobiologist Michael Merzenich of the University of California, San Francisco. "But a flood of discoveries shows that the brain continuously reorganizes itself."

"It's called neuroplasticity, and it means that you create the brain from the input you get," says Paula Tallal, co-director for the Center for Molecular and Behavioral Neuroscience at Rutgers University in New Jersey. "This means that your brain can produce new cells, or neurons. Scientists once thought that once you lost the brain cells, they were gone forever, but that's no longer the case."

It's a simple formula: increased firing (impulse) = increased brain cells = increased health. In future chapters of this book, I will explain to you how to increase the firing of your brain cells, or neuroplasticity.

Increased impulses, frequencies of firing, neuroplasticity or whatever you would like to call it can be proven objectively simply be re-testing (see Chapter 4 Examination) the patient following a specific treatment. If the test improved, the treatment worked. If the test did not improve or became worse, that is obviously not the treatment choice. Because of the speed with which the nervous system operates, objective neurological changes can happen very quickly; sometimes in an instant.

Your brain has a somatotopic map of the body super-imposed on it. If you look at the first picture (figure 3-4), the gray area in the picture below is the motor strip.

If I take a cross-section of the motor strip and look at one side of the hemisphere (bottom picture in Figure 3-4), you can see where

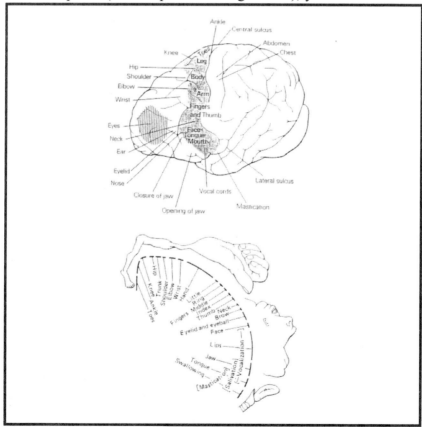

Figure 3-4

the leg is in the central portion. Observe how large of an area the face and the hand have in the overall representation. Notice the small representation of the lower back. Do you wonder why 80 million people suffer with lower back and leg pain? Because the lower back has such a small representation on the somatotopic map, it will have a decreased number of impulses in that area to begin with. If the impulses, or firing, are decreased over time because of stress, lower back pain will likely develop. Lower impulses equals increased pain!

The brain also contains the cerebellum (figure 3-5). The cerebellum controls balance and coordinated movement. It controls all of the spinal postural muscles and terminates eye movement. The brainstem, another part of the brain, is composed of three portions: top, middle, and lower. (figure 3-6) Of course, neurologists can't just use *top*, *middle*, and *lower*, but they have to use big, fancy words. And they can't just use one big, fancy word - they need to use several big, fancy words to describe one neuro-anatomical area. The top part of the brainstem is called the mesen-cephalon, also known as the midbrain or cerebral peduncle. The middle part, where the bulge is located, is called the pons, and the lower third is called the medulla oblongata. The two lower regions work together and are called the ponto-medullary region.

Under normal conditions, the brain fires impulses down to the lower two-thirds of the brainstem, or ponto-medullary area. The

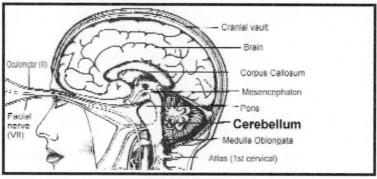

Figure 3-5

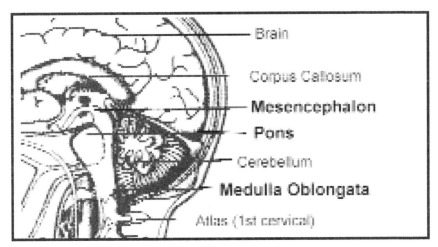

Brain
Corpus Callosum
Mesencephalon
Pons
Cerebellum
Medulla Oblongata
Atlas (1st cervical)

Figure 3-6

ponto-medullary area inhibits, or slows, the mesencephalon, the top portion of the brainstem. When there is a lack of firing down to the ponto-medullary area (lower brainstem), there is a failure to inhibit the mesencephalic output (upper brainstem). Usually, if a patient has a high-firing mesencephalon, he will be light-sensitive. He will either be very warm or very cold all of the time and will sweat very easily. He may also notice that his heart races. The heart contains two electrical nodes that allow it to beat: the SA node on the right and the AV node on the left (figure 3-7). The mesencephalon also drives down the spinal cord to an organ called the adrenal medulla. The adrenal medulla (figure 3-8) will release chemicals, called nor-epinephrine and catecholamines, into the blood that stimulate small nerve fibers. These small nerve fibers are pain fibers, called noci-ceptive or type-C fibers. Also with a high firing mesencephalon, the patient will have difficulty going to the bathroom. Control of the bowels and the ability to urinate are all conditions that can be treated by a chiropractic neurologist. The lower 2/3 of the brain-stem, called the ponto-medullary region, normally inhibits the upper region, the mesencephalon. The ponto-medullary area allows you to go to the bathroom, and the mesencephalon stops you

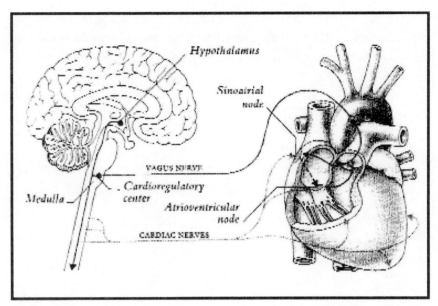

Figure 3-7

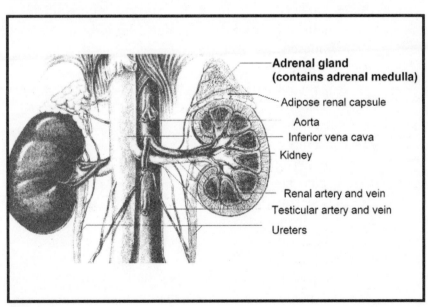

Figure 3-8

from going to the bathroom. If you increase the firing to the ponto-medullary area, (lower brainstem) you go, and if you increase the firing to the mesencephalon, (upper brainstem) you don't.

Chapter 4:
Examination

Before I treat any patient, I perform a comprehensive examination; for me to do anything less would be a grave disservice to the patient. No single test can specifically diagnose a condition. All tests, along with the patient's case history, must be considered to make a clinical diagnosis. I pride myself in providing one of the most complete and thorough neurological examinations in the country. The following is an example of my examination and the purpose of each test:

Blood Pressure
Blood pressure is taken on both sides of the body, or bilaterally. Normal blood pressure is around 120-130/80-90. The side that is measured higher may indicate the side of decreased brain function. The ponto-medullary region lowers the blood pressure, and the mesencephalon, or upper brainstem, raises blood pressure. When a patient has a decrease in frequency of firing of the brain, the brain will fail to stimulate the ponto-medullary region, which will fail to inhibit, or slow, the mesencephalon. The increased firing of the mesencephalon causes the patient's blood pressure to increase.

SpO2
Tissue saturation of oxygen is checked bilaterally and it measures the amount of oxygen in the patient's system. SpO2, or tissue saturation of oxygen, should ideally measure 98-100%. Tissue, especially brain tissue, needs oxygen as fuel to survive. Many medical doctors say that a tissue saturation of oxygen above 90% is fine. This is acceptable when examining a patient's cardiovascular output, but when observing the neurological stamina of the patient, the optimal saturation of oxygen must be considered.

Note: We check a patient's blood pressure, pulse, and tissue saturation of oxygen before and after each treatment. If I am truly stimulating brain function, the blood pressure and pulse should stay the same or decrease after each treatment because stimulation of the brain will cause increased firing into the lower brainstem.

Respiration
Respiration should measure 9-12 full breaths per minute. If the respiratory rate is above twelve breaths per minute, the patient is hyperventilating, which may indicate that the brainstem is overfiring. A respiratory rate of less than eight breaths per minute may not deliver enough oxygen to body tissue.

Pulse
A normal pulse rate should measure between 65 – 75 beats per minute.

Salivary pH
Optimum salivary pH is 7.0. A pH below 7.0 may indicate a decrease in tissue saturation of oxygen.

Chest Expansion
Chest expansion is measured during one complete breath cycle. A minimum chest expansion is 3 inches for females and 4 inches for males. Decreased chest expansion may indicate a decrease in exchange of air due to a decrease in lung tidal volume, possible rib interference, or lung disease.

Urinalysis and Blood Work
On every patient, I request a urinalysis to check the consistency, content, and color of the urine. A number of different conditions can be detected through urinalysis. I also request a complete blood work-up consisting of a complete blood chemistry, a complete metabolic panel, and a lipid panel. If the patient has had these tests performed by a medical doctor in the last three months, I will review the results when I request the patient's records. I recently had a patient who was in her mid-forties present to my office with lower back pain. After a six-week treatment, her pain would continually decrease and increase. Finally, I decided to obtain a blood work-up and urinalysis because she had not had these tests performed for some time. Her blood chemistry came back positive for a high sed-rate. A high sed-rate meant that she could have just about anything. The rest of her blood work, along with the urinalysis, was clean. The medical doctor I was working with at the time decided to obtain a lumbar spine MRI that came back negative. We then decided to get a cervical spine MRI due to the possibility of spinal cord compression in the cervical spine causing the pain. This also came back negative. Finally, we decided to obtain an

MRI of the patient's brain. Sure enough, this patient had a benign brain tumor that was causing her back pain. We immediately referred her to a neurosurgeon. There are old sayings in healthcare like "anything can cause anything" and "when you hear hoof beats, think of horses, not zebras," meaning that when a patient presents to your office with lower back pain, don't think of a brain tumor, but start with the simplest diagnosis and work your deferential diagnosis from there.

Finger Tip Glucose
Non-fasting finger-tip glucose testing is a screening test to measure levels of glucose in the blood. Glucose and oxygen are the two primary sources of fuel for the brain.

Muscle Stretch Reflexes (figure 4-1)
Biceps, triceps, brachioradialis and patellar should be +2 on both sides, meaning that when the doctor taps the reflexes the arm or leg should bounce. A decrease in reflexes indicates decreased brain function of the opposite brain hemisphere. Hyper-reflexes, or too much bounce, may also indicate decreased brain function of the opposite hemisphere.

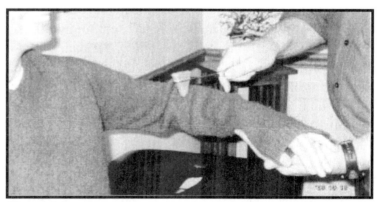

Figure 4-1

Vibratory Sensation (figure 4-2)

Vibratory sensation should be perceived equally on both sides of the body. Vibration tests the back part of the spinal cord, known as the dorsal column. Decreased vibratory sense on one side may indicate decreased brain function of the same or opposite hemisphere, depending on the correlation of other findings.

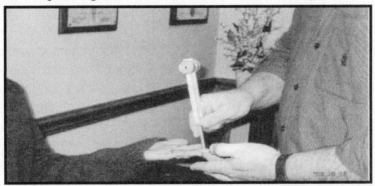

Figure 4-2

Pinwheel Sensation (figure 4-3)

The pinwheel is used to test pain sensation and compare the feeling from side to side. Pinwheel testing on the upper and lower extremities, face, or chest tests the front part of the spinal cord. Decreased sensation on one side can indicate decreased brain function of the same or opposite hemisphere, depending on a correlation of other findings.

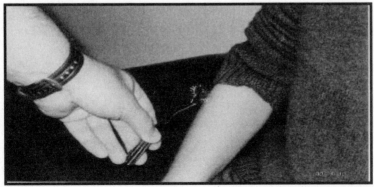

Figure 4-3

Muscle Strength

Muscle strength is tested to compare strength side to side. Decreased muscle strength on one side may indicate decreased brain function on the same or opposite side, depending upon a correlation of other findings.

Ear Exam
Weber

A tuning fork is placed on the top of the head; the patient should be able to hear the sound equally in both ears. Sound that occurs louder in one ear than the other (lateralization) may reveal cerumen (ear wax) blocking the ear canal or a nerve conduction problem.

Rinne

A tuning fork is held on bone behind the ear (mastoid) until the sound is no longer heard. The tuning fork is then placed in front of the ear canal. Air conduction (sound in front of the ear) should be heard after bone conduction (sound of the mastoid) ceases. If the patient cannot hear the sound in front of the ear, hearing may be blocked due to wax or nerve damage.

Visual Ear Exam

The external ear canal should be clear with no wax or redness observed. The eardrum (tympanic membrane) should be pearly gray in color and should reflect light. Infections of the inner or middle ear can cause a change in the eardrum color or size.

Eye Exam (figure 4-4)

The eyes are inspected for equal size, shape, overall appearance, and position. Difference from side to side may indicate decreased brain function, when correlated with other findings.

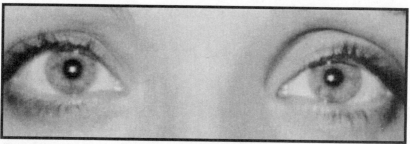

Figure 4-4

Corneal Reflex – Cranial Nerves #5 and #7 (figure 4-5)

Checking the corneal reflex cranial nerve #5 (sensation) and cranial nerve #7 (eye closure). The patient is asked to move the eye to one side and look up. A puff of air or piece of tissue touches the eye. The eye should blink reflexively and the sensation should be perceived equally in both eyes. If the eye doesn't blink equally, cranial nerve #7 may have decreased output on that side. Decreased sensation may indicate decreased function of cranial nerve #5 on that same side.

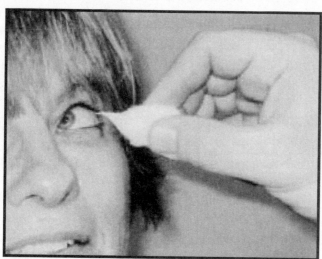

Figure 4-5

Corneal Light Reflection

The corneal light reflection is tested by shining a light at the bridge of the nose and observing the reflection. The eyes should remain neutral, not deviating in or out from neutral. If one eye deviates from the midline, it may indicate decreased brain function when correlated with other findings.

Pupillary Reflex - Cranial Nerve #3 (direct and indirect)
The pupillary reflex is tested by shining a light into the eye and observing the pupil becoming smaller. A slow response or even bouncing (hippus) may indicate decreased brain function. When the light is removed, the pupil should become larger.

Accommodation - Cranial Nerve #3
The patient is told to watch an object as it is brought in towards the nose. The eyes should converge toward the nose. If one eye moves out, this may indicate decreased brain function of that same side.

Pupil Size - Cranial Nerve #3 (figure 4-6)
Pupil size should be equal side to side. A larger pupil (corectasia) may indicate decreased brain function on that same side.

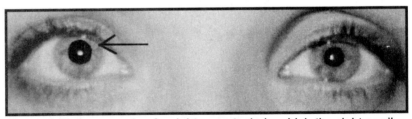

Figure 4-6 An example of a right corectasia in which the right pupil is larger than the left

Rapid Eye Movement Between Two Specific Points

The patient looks from one finger at midline to finger in the periphery as quickly as possible. Decreased speed or coordination when moving to one side may indicate decreased cerebellar function on the opposite side or decreased brain function on same side.

Cover/Uncover Test

The patient fixates gaze on a distant point, and vision in one eye is blocked by holding thumb over one pupil and taking away quickly. The eyes are observed for any deviation from normal position. Abnormal motion of either eye can indicate decreased brain function on that side.

Ocular Motion - Cranial Nerves #3, 4, and 6

Ocular motion is checked while the eyes follow an object through different visual fields. Muscle weakness or vibration of the eye is noted. Any decreased ocular motion may indicate decreased brain function of that side. Eye braking, or termination of movement, is also considered at the end of each visual field. Decreased braking may indicate decreased cerebellar function.

Peripheral Vision

A patient's peripheral vision is compared side to side. Differences from side to side can involve decreased brain function of either side when compared with other findings.

V/A Ratio

V/A ratio stands for the vein to artery ratio in the eye. The ratio should be 1:1 in each eye. A higher vein to artery ratio in one eye may indicate higher blood pressure on that side, indicating decreased brain function.

Optokinetic Tape (figure 4-7)

The patient follows a red and white tape with his/her eyes. Decreased movement on one side indicates decreased function of the parietal and frontal lobes of brain (on that side) or decreased cerebellar function on the opposite side, depending on eye movement.

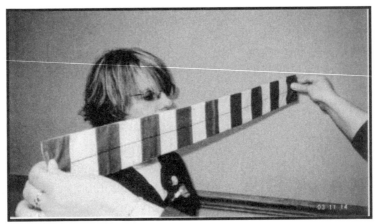

Figure 4-7

Blind Spot Mapping (figure 4-8)

The patient is asked to cover one eye and observe the red tip on a white pencil with his/her peripheral vision. The pencil is moved from the black dot, and when the red tip disappears from view, the area is marked. Once all areas are outlined, a comparison is made side to side, looking for similarity in shape (no irregularities), size (smaller than a quarter), and regularity from top to bottom. Differences in characteristics indicate decreased brain function on the opposite side.

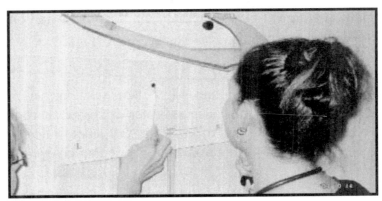

Figure 4-8

Olfactory Testing - Cranial Nerve #1
Olfactory testing is the difference in the ability to smell from side to side. Decreased smell on one side indicates decreased brain function on that side.

Facial Muscles - Cranial Nerve # 7
All facial muscles should look the same on both sides while smiling, wrinkling the forehead, biting down, and frowning. A decreased tone on one side of the face indicates decreased brain function on the same side or opposite side, depending on other findings.

Cranial Nerve #11
The cranial nerve #11 allows the patient to move his head from side to side and shrug his shoulders. Differences side to side can indicate a lesion in cranial nerve #11.

Cranial Nerve #12
When testing cranial nerve #12, the tongue should protrude in the midline. A tremor or deviation to one side may indicate a problem with the 12th cranial nerve.

Testing the Cerebellum
Romberg's Sign (figure 4-9)
The patient stands with both feet together and eyes closed. The patient should stand tall without sway. Swaying back and forth or falling to one side indicates decreased cerebellar function.

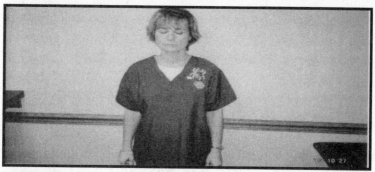

Figure 4-9

Arm Slap (figure 4-10)

The patient stands with both feet together and eyes closed. Hands are straight and outstretched. The examiner pushes the arm toward the floor. The patient's arm should return quickly to its initial position. Overshooting the original position can indicate decreased cerebellum function on that same side.

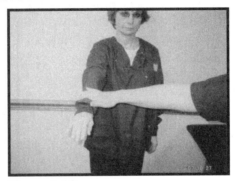

Figure 4-10

Past Pointing (figure 4-11)

The patient stands with feet together, eyes closed, and hands out in front. He/She should be able to touch his/her finger to his/her nose without difficulty. Missing the nose or ratchety motion when moving toward the nose may indicate decreased cerebellar function on that same side.

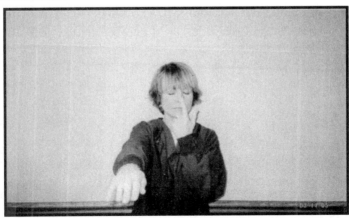

Figure 4-11

Piano (figure 4-12)

The patient is asked to pretend to play the piano with his/her arms straight out in front of him/her. Rapid and equal motion should be present in both hands. Decreased motion in one hand may indicate decreased cerebellar function on that side.

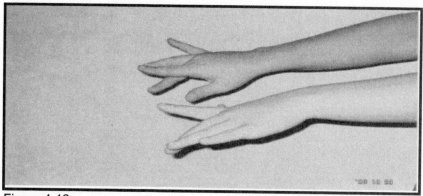

Figure 4-12

Supination/Pronation (figure 4-13)

The patient quickly turns his/her hands up (supination) and down (pronation). Speed and coordination should be equal in both hands. Decreased speed or coordination in one hand may indicate decreased cerebellar function on that side.

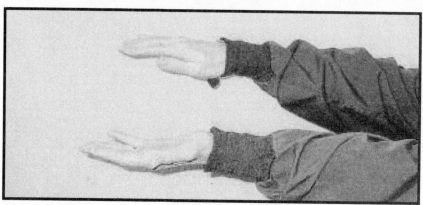

Figure 4-13

Heel Tap (figure 4-14)

The patient places one heel over the other shin and taps the shin with the heel as rapidly as possible on the same spot. Uncoordinated tapping may indicate decreased cerebellar function on that same side.

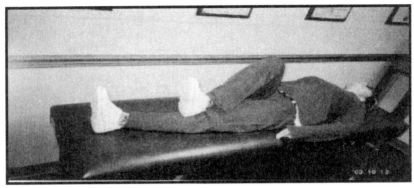

Figure 4-14

Heel to Toe Walk (figure 4-15)

The patient walks in a straight line with the heel touching the toe on every step. Any unsteadiness in gait may indicate decreased function on one side.

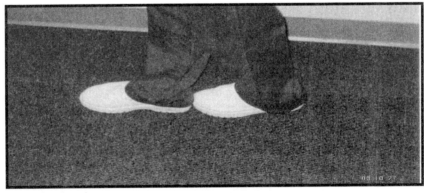

Figure 4-15

Running Heel Down Shin (figure 4-16)

Beginning at the knee and moving down to the ankle, the patient moves the heel down the opposite shin. The motion should be smooth and coordinated with both feet. Ratchety motion on one side can indicate a problem with the outside of the cerebellum on that same side.

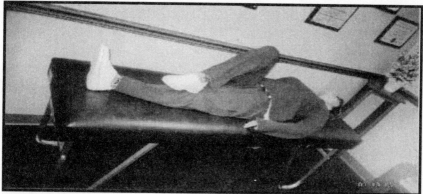

Figure 4-16

Windshield Wiper Blades
The lower extremities are tested by moving both feet in a wind-shield wiper pattern. The pattern should be smooth and at the same speed on both sides of the body. Decreased speed in one foot can indicate decreased outside cerebellar function on that side.

Temporal Lobe (figure 4-17)

Repeat Numbers
The patient should be able to repeat seven numbers back to the examiner. The inability to repeat the numbers spoken in a mono-tone voice indicates decreased left temporal lobe function, and the inability to repeat numbers spoken in a rhythmic variation indicates decreased right temporal lobe function.

Parietal Lobe (figure 4-17)
Parietal Sway
The patient stands with feet together, eyes closed, and hands

44

straight out in front. If one arm drifts away from original position, a parietal lobe soft lesion should be suspected.

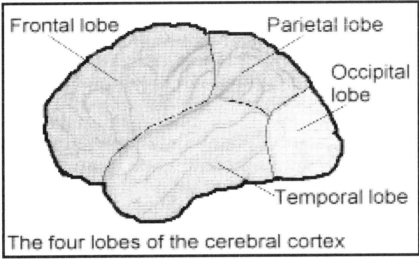

Figure 4-17

Two-Point Discrimination
Two-point discrimination should be distinguishable between two separate areas of the body, including the left side from the right while the patient's eyes are closed.

Heart Exam
A heart exam is performed by listening to the patient's heart for any abnormal sounds, such as clicks or gallops. Rhythm is also noted in the form of normal rhythm (sinus rhythm) or uneven rhythm (arrhythmia). Uneven rhythm may indicate a decreased left brain function. Heart rate is also noted. A normal heart rate is measured at 60-100 beats per minute. Fast heart beats (over 100) equal tachycardia, while slow beats (under 60) equal bradycardia. Either tachycardia or bradycardia may indicate a decreased right brain function.

Abdominal Exam
The exam is performed by listening to bowel sounds in the four dif-

ferent areas, or quadrants, of the abdomen. Bowel sounds should be heard in each area within 10 seconds. Decreased bowel sounds could indicate a bowel obstruction and further testing is warranted. Pressure is applied to the same four areas of the abdomen looking for pain, lumps or bumps. Tapping over all four quadrants is also performed with any difference in sound noted. Aerophagia (the swallowing of air) can be heard as a hollow sound over one or more of the four quadrants.

Bruits
The examiner listens to the blood vessels in the head, neck, and abdomen for blood vessel narrowing.

Orthopedic Exams
Several orthopedic exams are performed on each patient. The purpose of orthopedic tests is to identify problems within certain areas of the body. Groups of tests focus on diagnoses for different regions of the body. The areas are divided into neck (cervical), mid-back (thoracic), low back (lumbopelvic), and extremity.

ROM
Range of Motion is performed in different areas of the spine. Cervical (neck), thoracic (chest), lumbar and pelvic (low back) areas are all considered. Base-line degrees of motion are expected and decreased motion in one or more can indicate joint fixation, sprain-strain, or other pathology.

Posture
The patients overall posture is observed. A high shoulder, head tilt, high hip or weight bearing are noted. Gait is also analyzed. Patterns of movement during walking may be observed. Movement can give clues to assess overall brain function.

Re-Examination
A re-exam will be performed at specific interim points of care. This

re-exam will check whether progress has been made to date and identify areas needing more work.

It is all well and good that a patient's subjective findings improve (symptoms get better), but symptomatic changes can happen as a result of a placebo effect. How do I truly know that I have made a positive change in a patient's nervous system? The re-examination provides me with that information. Did the patient's exphoria (eye popping out), corectasia (large pupil), palatal paresis, Romberg's sign, pupillary reflex, or optokinetic tape test improve? If it did, then I know that I have made a positive change that can be proven objectively. My patients may want symptomatic change, but I look for objective results.

Chapter 5:
Treatment Modalities

"Our prayers should be for a sound
mind in a healthy body."
-Juvenal: *Satires*, Satire, X

I never prescribe a treatment without first performing a compre-hensive neurological exam. All of the treatment modalities are closely monitored by pre- and post-blood pressure, pulse, and neu-rological testing. Increased frequency of firing of the cortex (increasing brain function) should maintain or lower the blood pressure and pulse via the neo-cortico-thalamo-hypothalamo-ponto-medullary reticular activating system. See what I mean about big words? I just think it's fun to say. The following are examples of the latest, state-of-the-art treatment protocols, all scientifically based and referenced:

Unilateral Manipulation

The extremities (knee, ankle, wrist, elbow), lower back, and neck may be adjusted. Joint manipulation (structural adjustments) is only performed on one side of the body to increase brain function of the opposite cortex (brain) and ipsilateral, or same-side, cerebellum (back part of the brain). At each visit, objective findings will assist in determining what regions of the spine will be adjusted, and these may vary from appointment to appointment. Lower frequency modalities, including activators, may be used. With an activator, a hand-held instrument, the practitioner can administer a very low-force adjustment to a particular vertebra. The activator is very beneficial to people suffering from migraine headaches, fibromyalgia, and dizziness. (See page 72 for an explanation of an indepth manipulation.)

Dorsal Spine Adjustment: Thoracic adjustment to activate dorsal column pathways, to increase tidal volume of lungs, and to address subluxation concerns.

Upper Extremity Adjustment: Utilizing muscle spindle afferents (large diameter 1A afferents, i.e. large nerves) in the wrist and elbow to stimulate the cuneocerebellar tract that activates the fastigium within the ipsilateral (same side) cerebellum, then is a feed-forward (cerebellum to brain) mechanism to the opposite brain.

Lower Extremity Adjustment: Utilizing muscle spindle afferents (i.e. large nerves) in the ankle and lateral knee to stimulate the spinocerebellar tract to activate the fastigium within the ipsilateral cerebellum, that is a feed-forward mechanism to the opposite brain.

Auditory Stimulation (Appendix II)

Auditory stimulation in one ear is utilized to increase the firing, or impulses, of the opposite cortex (temporal lobe of the brain) via the inferior colliculus (appendix II) of the mesencephalon (top part of the brainstem). Blood pressure, pulse, and neurological findings before and after treatment determine the type and length of treatment at each visit. Auditory stimulation will vary from 1-20 minutes per treatment.

Metronome: The metronome works well when both the cerebellum and the brain need to be stimulated with a low metabolic demand. The metronome beats can range from 40 beats per minute to 74 beats per minute, but the rate should not exceed the patient's heart rate.

Rain/thunderstorm: Nature sounds stimulate the opposite cortex and usually work well in patients with hypertension, or high blood pressure.

Mozart: Mozart in a major key stimulates the opposite cortex. The major key has a higher metabolic demand than other forms of auditory stimulation, and it should therefore be used judiciously.

Visual Stimulation (Appendix II)

Watching a checkerboard pattern can increase brain function when viewed in only one-half or one-quarter of a patient's visual field. Visual stimulation coming from the left visual field crosses through the superior colliculus in the upper brainstem, which increases activation in the cerebral cortex, or right-brain. Increased activity of the brain should lower the blood pressure and pulse via the ponto-medullary (lower brainstem) stimulation. The intensity of treatment can be varied by using different color combinations. Frequency varies by rate of color and the various checkerboard patterns. Color frequencies from lowest to highest are red/black, red/green, blue/black, and light blue/dark blue. Frequency (speed of movement) can range from 2-8 Hz.

A red or green light may be shown in the nasal aspect of the right or left eye. This increases the activity of the superior colliculus of the opposite mesencephalon, or upper brainstem, to reduce the activation of the mesencephalic reticular activating system (ex. lower pulse). Remember that the mesencephalic reticular activating system is simply the brain firing to lower brainstem. Apparently, it's too easy for neurologists to state that the brain fires to the lower brainstem, so they need to call it neo-cortical-thalamo-hypothalamo-mesencephalic reticular activating system.

Faces: The act of viewing pictures of faces increases brain function via a feed-forward mechanism through the cerebellum to the cortex. Faces specifically stimulate the amygdala, which lies deep in the temporal lobe. The amygdala is the rapid response system of the body. It sends the body into a high alert if triggered. Usually, the front part of the brain, called the prefrontal cortex, controls the amygdala. In people who suffer from an anxiety or phobia, the prefrontal cortex may lose its ability to control the amygdala, allowing the amygdala to cause fear in unthreatening situations. The amygdala also recognizes faces. Familiar faces will stimulate the left amygdala, and unfamiliar faces will stimulate the right.

Eye exercises: Eye exercises will increase activation into the cerebellum. The lateral cortex of the cerebellum will be activated and will improve connections to the contralateral, or opposite, frontal cortex (front part of the brain).

Mazes/Word Searches: (Appendix II) Mazes will activate the right parietal lobe, and word searches will activate the left parietal lobe.

Large Letters Made of Small Letters: (Appendix II) Observing only the large letters will stimulate the right hemisphere, or right-brain. Observing only the small letters will stimulate the left hemisphere, or left-brain.

T.E.N.S.
T.E.N.S. stands for Transcutaneous Electronic Nerve Stimulation. Electrical stimulation is used at a subthreshold level (the patient cannot feel it) to decrease pain sensation and increase the function of the opposite hemisphere (brain) and the same-side cerebellum. Since the right-brain controls the left side of the body and the left-brain controls the right side of the body, T.E.N.S. should be administered to the opposite brain area (left side for right-brain). Normal brain frequency is 8-13 Hz, so the T.E.N.S. frequency is set in this range.

Heat
Heat therapy is used to promote an increase metabolic and healing rate to the involved tissue. Increased heat increases the activation to the brain. Heat has an immediate soothing effect, decreasing joint stiffness and muscle spasms by increasing the frequency of firing of the cerebellum and brain. Ice decreases frequency of firing or impulses to the brain.

Ultrasound
Ultrasound is utilized to provide a deep, muscular vibratory sensation to increase the vascular supply to the involved tissue.

Intersegmental Traction
Intersegmental traction is performed on a mechanical table, and it increases vibration into the dorsal column, the back part of the spinal cord. This form of vibration activates the patient's proprioceptive system (tells the brain where the body is in space). The dorsal column fires up to the cerebellum, increasing the cerebellar frequency of firing.

Warm and Cold Calorics

Placing warm water or air in the ear stimulates the cerebellum on the same side via the semicircular canal of the ear and the vestibular nerve (figure 5-1). The warm water stimulates the semicircular canals by increasing the flow of the endolymph. Endolymph is a gelatinous material that resembles Jell-O. Everyone knows that when you warm up Jell-O, it liquefies. When the endolymph is warmed to a higher temperature, the endolymph becomes liquefied and stimulates hair cells in the semicircular canals called stereocillia and kinocillia. The stereocillia and kinocillia fire, or excite, the vestibular nerve back to the cerebellum, and they therefore increase the frequency of firing, or impulses, to the same side cerebellum. Cold or ice calorics may be used to diagnose a particular condition. When ice water is placed in the ear, the exact opposite effect of a

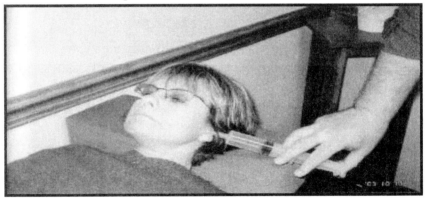

Figure 5-1

warm caloric is initiated. The endolymph would be more gelatin-like and would fail to stimulate the stereocilia and kinocilia. The same side cerebellum would have a decreased frequency of firing, allowing the practitioner to test the neuroplasticity, or function, of the opposite cerebellum. Calorics are very helpful in the treatment of vertigo/dizziness.

UBE

The UBE, or Upper Body Ergometer, is like an exercise bike for the arms. The UBE will increase the firing of the posterior muscle groups, neck, and arms to fire the cuneo-cerebellar tract bilaterally to the cerebellum, increasing its activation. The UBE will also activate the muscles of posture. The arms (cuneo-cerebellar tract) fire much more powerfully to the cerebellum than the legs (spino-cerebellar). For this reason, I always recommend exercising with the UBE over the treadmill. Personally, I use my UBE daily for 30 minutes.

Olfactory Stimulation

Olfactory stimulation (stimulating smell) through one nostril is used to increase the frequency of firing, or impulses, to the temporal lobe of the same-side brain.

Visual Imagery

Visual imagery entails imaging one's body going through certain motions. Depending on head position, this will stimulate the semicircular canals of the ear and will activate brain function.

Eye Exercises

Eye exercises slow to the right will engage the parietal cortex with a fast saccade back to the left engaging the right frontal cortex and the contralateral or left cerebellum terminates the eye movement.

Mirror Imagery

The patient observes one-half of the body in the mirror. This half will be moved to project that the opposite side of the body, the side that is not working, is also moving. Mirror imagery increases the frequency of firing of the brain via activation of the somatotopic map. Mirror imaging is especially helpful in stroke rehabilitation where the patient has lost the use of one side of the body.

Spin Therapy
Spinning a patient at a slow to moderate rate in a clockwise or counter-clockwise direction stimulates the semicircular canals (see Figure 6-1, page 59) in much the same way as a caloric by increasing the flow of the endolymph. The endolymph excites the stereocillia and kinocillia that excite the vestibular nerve and increase the frequency of firing of the same-side cerebellum. Spinning to the right increases the impulses to the right cerebellum, and spinning to the left increases the impulses to the left cerebellum.

Oxygen
Supplemental oxygen will be given to patients to increase the vascular supply, or fuel, to brain tissues. Oxygen is fuel for the brain, the brainstem, and especially the cerebellum. The cerebellum is the most oxygen-dependent organ in the body. The brain requires two things to survive: fuel, in the form of oxygen and glucose, and activation. The brain receives glucose from food and oxygen from the air. Movement, along with many of the previous treatment modalities, causes activation. The normal inspiration/expiration ratio of an individual should be 1:2, meaning that you should breathe out twice as long as you breathe in. When a patient suffers from a low tissue saturation of oxygen, I will often assign this breathing exercise.

Ultimate Eye Filters
A decreased frequency of firing from the brain down to the lower brainstem, or ponto-medullary area, causes an increase in the frequency of firing of the upper brainstem, the mesencephalon. As a result of the high frequency of firing of the upper brainstem, the patient's pupil will dilate and the patient will experience some or all of the following symptoms: light sensitivity, increased perspiration, rapid heart rate, increased warmth, and chronic pain syndromes. These symptoms are created when the mesencephalon (upper brainstem) drives down the spinal cord, causing a release of pain-producing chemicals. Light and sound are the two most powerful

stimulants to the upper brain stem. I developed the *Ultimate Eye Filters* to decrease the wavelength of light entering the patient's brainstem. Let me give you an example: if you spray Windex on your television or computer monitor you will see three colors - red, green, and blue - yet on the television you will see the entire spectrum of color. White light is primarily composed of these three wavelengths. White light is the highest frequency, blue light the next highest, green light slightly lower, and red light the lowest. *Ultimate Eye Filters* are a patented technology that decreases the wavelength of light entering the upper brainstem, or mesencephalon. By slowing down the firing of the upper brainstem and increasing the firing of the lower brainstem, the pupil will become smaller and the upper brainstem will decrease in the frequency of firing. A decrease in the frequency of firing of the upper brainstem will cause a constriction of the blood vessels in the brain, and this in turn will help relieve a patient's migraine headaches, light sensitivity and overall firing into the upper brainstem.

Millions of people work in front of computer monitors every day. Even with a glare filter on a computer monitor, it is necessary to utilize the *Ultimate Eye Filters* because the technology decreases the frequency of light into the brainstem itself.

What can I do to help myself?

I get this question from every patient. Why? Because they want to get better as fast as possible. Therefore, I've included the following list:

Squeezeball (to increase the impulses to the cerebellum)

Backstroke (pretend you are swimming the backstroke for 3 minutes twice a day, this also increases impulses to the cerebellum.

Spinning (see spin therapy)

Faces

Mazes (see mazes)

UBE (located at most YMCA's and health clubs)

Olfactory stimulation (very powerful-so be careful)

Auditory stimulation (many tapes are available)

Big letters made up of small letters

Heat

Mirror imagery (if the patient had suffered a stroke)

All of these can be utilized to increase brain frequency of firing or impulses. Start slow, perhaps one or two, and add others as you go along.

If problems arise, consult a board certified chiropractic neurologist @ www.DACNB.org. Ideally, I recommend that you consult a chiropractic neurologist first!

Chapter 6:
Vertigo/Dizziness

"Say you are well, or all is well with you,
and God shall hear your words and make them true."
-Ella Wheeler Wilcox: *Speech*,
Rand McNally & Co.

According to the Vestibular Disorders Association, vertigo and dizziness affect millions of people around the world each year. More than 90 million adult Americans have experienced a dizziness or balance problem, and 40% of the population over age 40 will suffer from a dizziness disorder in their lifetime. Balance disorder is one of the two most common diagnoses among short-stay hospital admissions in individuals over the age of 65. Balance-related falls account for more than half the accidental deaths and 75% of emergency room visits of the elderly population. The cost of medical care for patients with balance disorders exceeds $1 billion yearly in the U.S. alone. More than 5 million Americans visited their doctors in 1995 because of vertigo. The disability was so severe in an estimated 10% of these patients that they had to be hospitalized. In the last 10 years, diagnosis and treatment of vestibular disorders has changed dramatically. Many other symptoms may now be associated with vertigo, including trouble writing, trouble reading, and visual changes. These visual changes may include poor depth perception, increased night blindness, or sensitivity to moving or flickering lights. In many vertiginous patients, hearing may fluctuate, and the patient may hear a popping, clicking, buzzing, or ringing in the ears. The patient's ears may also have a "full feeling" due to blockage of the Eustachian tube. Many times, patients will be diagnosed with Meniere's Syndrome, a combination of dizziness, loss of hearing, and tinnitus (ringing in the ears). Nausea, intermittent nausea, or motion sickness may accompany dizziness in many cases. Coordination may be affected; patients may be clumsier or may veer to one side when walking. Memory may be very poor, and patients may forget words that they are about to say. A vertiginous patient may also suffer from headaches, fatigue, and vomiting.

The two types of vertigo are called egocentric vertigo and geocentric vertigo. Geocentric vertigo means that the patient feels the room is spinning, and egocentric vertigo means that the patient feels they are spinning in the room. Patients may also suffer from light-headedness or episodic periods of dizziness.

The medical treatment of vertigo usually consists of the prescription of the medication Meclizine (dimenhydrinate). Every patient suffering from vertigo that I have treated has been on this medication at some point. It obviously did not work; if it did, they would not be in my office. I am sure that Meclizine has worked for some people, but those are the people who have not shown up at my door. In severe cases, the doctor may refer the patient to a physical therapist for canalith training, a series of head exercises.

Many medical diagnoses of vertigo include an "inner ear problem", which leads to a diagnosis of Benign Paroxysmal Positional

Vertigo (BPPV). Frankly, this is correct, but balance is also related to other neuro-anatomical areas which include the brain, (frontal lobe, basal ganglia, and cerebellum), spinal cord, visual system, and proprioceptors. If you remember earlier, I related how the cerebellum controls your balance and coordinated movement. Many times, after a thorough examination, I will find a decrease in the function of the right or left cerebellum. Then it is simply a matter of deciding which treatment modalities are best for the patient.

Your body contains many, many receptors. Light receptors in your eyes and sound receptors in your ears are two examples. The musculoskeletal system (arms, legs, back, and neck) has three specific receptors: muscle spindle cells (muscle receptors), joint-mechano receptors (receptors in joints), and golgi tendon organs (tendon receptors). These three receptor types fire different types of nerves into the spinal cord and up to the cerebellum. In technical jargon, "firing of 1A or 1B afferents via the spinal cerebellar tract up to the ipsilateral cerebellum." (See what I mean by doctors speaking in big terms to impress patients?) Sometimes the treatment consists of increasing the firing or impulses of these receptors via manipulation.

In this chapter, I provide examples of patients with vertigo or dizziness that have responded to the specific care that we provide in our offices. All of these patients had been under the care of numerous doctors and therapists without any relief. You will also notice the different types of treatment for each individual patient, a necessity that I cannot stress enough. Chiropractors are usually trained in one technique and will not deviate from that technique. In many cases, that technique may be too powerful for the individual patient, especially the vertigo patient. All of us have a baseline of our nervous system called the central integrated state, or CIS. When an adjustment or manipulation is administered, receptors are fired up the spinal cord to the same-side cerebellum. Therefore, you only want to utilize a unilateral, or one-sided, manipulation or adjustment.

A caloric may be used to treat a patient suffering from vertigo. A caloric, in the form of water or warm air into the ear, causes the endolymph, a gelatin-like substance inside the canals of the ear, to become warm and liquefy (see figure 6-1). The semicircular canals that contain endolymph also contain hair cells called stereocillia and kinocillia. When the endolymph is liquefied, it stimulates these hair cells, and when the hair cells are stimulated, they fire the vestibular nerve back to the cerebellum. By inducing warmth into

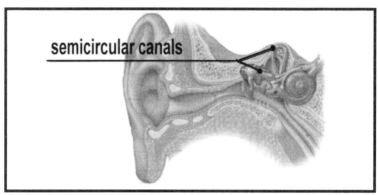

Figure 6-1

the ear canal, we increase the frequency of firing, or impulses, back to the cerebellum. The same is true with eye exercises. For instance, the right cerebellum controls eye movements up to the right, down to the left, and across to the left. The left cerebellum controls eye movements up to the left, down to the right, and across to the right. Therefore, I may incorporate eye exercises to relieve patients of vertigo.

Visual imagery is another treatment protocol that I have used with patients. In visual imagery, the patient imagines certain bodily movements to increase the frequency of firing to the cerebellum. As you will see the following cases, the imagery depends upon the patient's baseline of the nervous system, or central integrated state.

George
History:

One of my first patients with vertigo was a 67 year-old male named George. George had been suffering from vertigo for over five years. He had been on the medication Meclizine for some time and had previously been treated by a number of other chiropractors and medical doctors. He would often become so dizzy that he would vomit. Many patients vomit when they have migraines or dizziness because the lower brainstem (ponto-medullary area, figure 6-2) is overfiring. Inside this ponto-medullary area is another area called the NTS (Nucleus Tractus Solatarius) (figure 6-3), the area that emits the Vagus nerve (figure 6-4). The Vagus nerve is one of the nerves in the body that fires just about everywhere. It fires to the heart, the lungs, the large intestine, the pancreas, the liver, and the blood vessels in the abdomen. The Vagus nerve also fires to the gut, which is why people with dizziness and migraines may become nauseous.

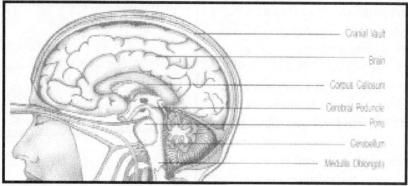

Figure 6-2

Examination:

Upon examination of George, I noted that his right pupil was enlarged which is indicative of a decrease in the firing of the right brain. I also found a decrease upon optokinetic tape testing to the right. An optokinetic tape is a red and white tape that allows the examiner to assess the frontal lobe, parietal lobe, and opposite cerebellum of the patient. In George's case, I found a decreased firing in the parietal lobe and frontal lobe on the right side. There was a marked decrease in muscle strength in both the upper and lower

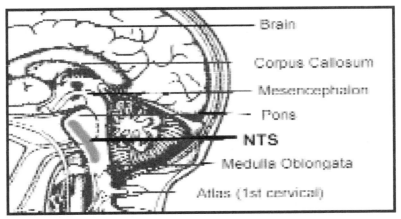

Figure 6-3

extremities. Upon testing Romberg's sign (standing with feet together and eyes closed) and Tandem walk (walking heel to toe), George exhibited a severe sway. Rapid hand acceleration, finger to nose, and past pointing were all decreased on the left. George had definite signs of a decreased firing, or impulses, in his right cortex and left cerebellum.

My treatment was manipulation on the right side of George's body. Manipulation fires joint receptors, muscle receptors, and tendon recep-

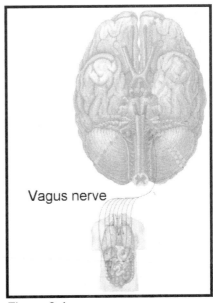

Figure 6-4

tors up the back part of the spinal cord to the same-side cerebellum. The first few treatments with George were very difficult. He would come into the office extremely dizzy and vomiting. After approximately four to five weeks, George was doing much better subjectively and objectively. And after twelve weeks, George no longer suffered from any symptoms of vertigo. I continue to treat George and his lovely wife Norma on a maintenance basis.

Rita
History:

Rita, a 68 year-old female, presented with severe geocentric vertigo. Geocentric vertigo, a condition where the patient feels as if the room is spinning, differs from egocentric vertigo, a condition where the patient feels that they are spinning. Usually, geocentric vertigo is much easier to treat than egocentric vertigo. Rita had suffered from this condition since 1963. Over the years, Rita had been treated by numerous medical doctors and had been on the medication Meclizine.

Examination:

Upon examination of Rita, I observed a severe right exophoria. When the examiner moves a pen toward the patient's nose, both eyes should converge. Rita exhibited a right exophoria in that her right eye would converge, and then pop out. This is indicative of a problem in the upper brainstem, since the fourth cranial nerve controls the convergence of the eyes. I also found a decrease in the optokinetic tape testing upon moving the tape to the right. Rita exhibited a severe sway upon testing Romberg's sign (standing with feet together and eyes closed) and Tandem walk (walking heel to toe). Past pointing and finger to nose testing were decreased on the left. I had Rita obtain a doppler study of the carotid arteries, since clotting within the carotid arteries can be a major cause of vertigo in the elderly. Fortunately for Rita, the doppler results were negative.

I treated Rita with manipulation on her left side to increase the frequency of firing, or impulses, of the left cerebellum. The left cerebellum is connected to the semicircular canals in the ear via the vestibular nerve, so I administered a warm caloric in the left ear to increase the movement of endolymph and excite the stereocilia and kinocilia (hair cells). Stimulation of these hair cells increases the frequency of firing (impulses) in the semicircular canals, firing the vestibular nerve back to the cerebellum. After ten weeks, Rita was completely free of dizziness or any vertiginous symptom. Objective findings had also improved. She no longer exhibited the right exophoria upon accomodation. Past pointing, finger to nose, Rhomberg's sign and optokinetic tape testing had also greatly improved. Forty years of suffering was eliminated with ten weeks of care. Wunderbar!

Barb
History:

Barb, a 61 year-old female, had been suffering from vertigo for four years. Barb had been treated by medical doctors, chiropractors, and physical therapists at the time she presented to my office, and she had been taking the medication Meclizine. I had originally treated Barb for a headache condition, and she obtained great results. Barb had been suffering from egocentric vertigo, feeling that she was spinning to her right. Again, from my experience, egocentric vertigo is much more difficult to treat then geocentric vertigo.

Examination:

Upon examination of Barb, I found many symptoms similar to other vertigo patients. She had an enlarged left pupil and a left exophoria, meaning that when she followed the pen to her nose, her left eye bounced out to the side. A decrease in the pupil response was also noticed. When the examiner shines a light into the pupil, the pupil should get smaller and stay smaller. In Barb's case, the pupil got smaller, then got bigger right away. The pupil then started bouncing, a condition called hippus. Barb exhibited a decrease in optokinetic tape testing when moving the optokinetic tape to the left. More specifically, I found a decrease in the firing of the left parietal lobe, left frontal lobe, and right cerebellum.

I also used an examination procedure called an electronystagographic examination. I use goggles similar to scuba goggles that contain a small infrared camera on one eye. When these goggles are placed on the patient, I can then observe and record the eye upon testing. When we had Barb look up and to her right, there was a sustained nystagmus, or a bouncing of the eyeball. I found that Barb suffered from transneural degeneration of the right cerebellum. Transneural degeneration occurs when neurons, or nerve cells, are dying off in the cerebellum, and before they die off, they fire at a very high rate.

I began a treatment protocol of adjusting Barb with an activator, a small hand-held instrument. I would only adjust Barb on her right side to increase impulses to her right cerebellum. I also used a warm caloric on the right side, similar to what I used with Rita. Upon utilizing these two treatment modalities, Barb became progressively worse, as I was exceeding her metabolic capacity. Finally, after further examination, I decided to prescribe eye exercises. Eye exercises will also increase the frequency of firing, or impulses, to the cerebellum. I had Barb follow a pen slowly up and to the right with her eyes. This action would fire the right parietal lobe and the right cerebellum. After this exercise, she would close her eyes, and when she reopened her eyes, she performed another slow pursuit up and to the right. This type of exercise would incorporate the anterior semicircular canal in the right ear. After one week of performing eye exercises, Barb's dizziness was completely resolved and objective examination findings had greatly improved, therefore I released her from care.

Char
History:

Char, a 32 year-old female, had suffered from severe vertigo for over five years. At the time of presentation, she was taking the drug Meclizine. Observing my patient population, I find that Meclizine is the #1 medication prescribed for dizziness. Although I have seen other medications utilized, Meclizine far exceeds any other type.

As usual, numerous medical doctors, chiropractors, and physical therapists had treated Char, and she stated to me that I was her "last resort" because I treat so many chronic patients. I hear that statement quite often.

Examination:

Upon examination, findings similar to those of other vertigo patients were noted. In addition, Char exhibited a sustained nystagmus up and to the right, meaning that when she looked up and to the right, her eyes were bouncing. Unfortunately for Char, every treatment modality that I utilized failed to provide any relief. Thankfully, after seeing so many other doctors, she decided to continue with treatment because I was at least trying new treatment modalities. Finally, after trying multiple treatment modalities with no avail, I went back and looked at the tape of the electronystagographic exam, the eye examination that we had initially performed on Char. I then decided to try visual imagery. Visual imagery is a feedback mechanism in which the patient imagines that she is floating, running, sitting, or standing. I had Char imagine that she was floating up and to her right, since the right cerebellum controls eye movement up and to the right, down and to the left, and over to the left. When she imagined floating up and to the right, her vertigo improved slightly. On her next visit, I told her to imagine that she was floating down and to her left. The minute she imagined that she was floating down and to the left, her vertigo subsided. I am very happy to report that Char has not suffered from vertigo since utilizing visual imagery in my office well over three years ago.

Esther
History:

Esther, a 63 year-old female, presented to my office complaining of severe vertigo, headaches, and chronic fatigue. She reported that her vertigo began one year before initiating treatment. She would experience dizziness on a daily basis with varying intensities. Esther reported that she also suffered from tachycardia (increased heart rate), light sensitivity, sleeplessness, and an increase in perspiration. These findings are indicative of an abnormally high-firing mesencephalon, or upper brainstem. Esther had stated that she had suffered a severe stroke in 1968, and as a result, she continued to experience a loss of grip strength and increasing weakness in her legs. She had completely lost her speech when she suffered the stroke, and she had to learn to speak again with the aid of a speech therapist. Esther stated that she could think of what she wanted to say, but she could not pronounce the words. This is a result of decreased firing of Broca's speech area (area #45) (figure 6-5), located in the left temporal lobe of the brain.

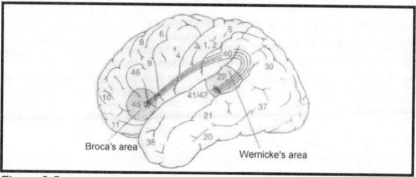

Figure 6-5

Examination:

Upon examining Esther, many positive findings were discovered, including a larger pupil on the left, a decreased pupillary reflex, a decrease in the optokinetic tape testing on the left, a facial paresis, and a palatal paresis on the left. When standing with her feet together and eyes closed, Esther exhibited a severe sway, indicative of a decrease in the frequency of firing of the cerebellum. Normally, the brain fires to the lower brainstem, the ponto-medullary area. The ponto-medullary region slows down, or inhibits, the upper brainstem. If the frequency of firing of the pathway from the brain to the lower brainstem is decreased, the mesencephalon, or upper brainstem, will fire at a very high rate and will cause all of symptoms that Esther was suffering from.

Esther was first treated with oxygen (per order of our medical doctor) via mask because her tissue saturation of oxygen was only 93%. She was also treated with a warm water caloric in her right ear to stimulate the right cerebellum. Warm water increases the frequency of firing, or impulses, of the semicircular canals into the ear (see figure B), which in turn will increase the frequency of firing of the same-side cerebellum via input from the vestibular nerve. Finally, unilateral manipulation was performed on the right side to further increase cerebellar firing. Due to the severity of Esther's case and the compromised metabolic rate of her nervous system, her case was extremely challenging. After her first eighteen-visit treatment trial, Esther showed a significant improvement. We re-examined Esther and found improvements both subjectively (symptoms) and objectively (exam findings). We then decided on another eighteen-visit treatment trial. Esther is just completing this treatment and is responding tremendously well both subjectively and objectively. She no longer has the constant dizziness, her overall energy has improved greatly, and she tells me that she feels like a new person!

(Please note that the preceding case histories are only a few of the thousands of patients that we have helped in our clinic in the past 20 years.)

Chapter 7:
Migraine Headaches

*"Look to your health; and if you have it, praise God,
and value it next to a good conscience; for health
is the second blessing that we mortals are capable of;
a blessing that money cannot buy."*
                                    -Isaac Walton: *Compleat Angler*,
                                                    Pt. I, ch. 21

I have a special affinity for migraine headache sufferers because I suffered from migraine headaches for over nine years. Many times, I would suffer from three serious migraines per week. Visual changes that looked like squiggly lines would begin in my left eye, and approximately twenty minutes after the aura change, an intense migraine would start. The intense pain felt like a spike was being driven through my left eye. In many instances, I would start vomiting after the migraine. Thankfully, in 1997, I discovered Dr. Carrick's work and got under the treatment of an associate. By using Dr. Carrick's techniques, I am happy to say that I have not suffered from a migraine headache since August 1998. When I am under intense stress, the aura (squiggly lines) may reappear, but these instances are rare.

Migraine headaches can be classified in two categories: classical and common. The classical migraine is a headache that follows an aura or some type of spontaneous event such as numbness or tingling, which is called a "prodrome" phase. The aura may be flashes of light, squiggly lines, or a halo effect. The common migraine does not have an aura associated with it. Most migraine headache sufferers suffer from common migraines, usually at a 3:1 ratio of classical to common. Approximately 28 million Americans suffer from migraine headaches, and millions go without treatment. Scientists once thought that migraines were caused by an abnormally dilated, or enlarged, blood vessel. New imaging devices have allowed them to observe the brain during migraine attacks, and scientists are discovering that migraine sufferers have abnormally excitable neurons, or brain nerve cells. The latest research concerning migraine headaches is a mechanism called cortical spreading depression, or CSD. Prior to the onset of the pain of a migraine, researchers have observed a sudden burst of cortical activity that occurs most commonly in the occipital lobes (back part of the brain). The occipital lobe will increase in the frequency of firing, or have a burst of activity; then it will have an episode of silence or depressed activity. The actual activity of the brain becomes depressed when compared to normal. The resulting pain comes from activation of the upper brainstem, or mesencephalon, which causes the blood vessels in the brain to become inflamed and then constrict very rapidly. An overfiring mesencephalon is also the reason why many patients experience an aura, whether it is a halo, squiggly lines, or some other type of visual disturbance.

I have treated hundreds of migraine sufferers. They are prescribed a litany of medications, including Imitrex (sumatriptan),

Topamax (topiramate), and even anti-seizure medications such as Klonopin (clonazepam). It's a Russian roulette of drug therapy. If this medication doesn't work, perhaps this one will. If that medication doesn't work, we'll try another. It's a revolving door, yet the patient continues to suffer.

I have found many cases where the medication benefits the patient initially, only to "wear off" over time. Initially, the medication works well and the symptoms abate, but over time, the medication fails and the symptoms return. My theory is that the brain habituates or "gets used to" the drug. The medication is a stimuli and the brain habituates to all stimuli.

As a board-certified chiropractic neurologist, specifically a Carrick-trained board-certified chiropractic neurologist, I take a different approach to the treatment and prevention of migraines. After a thorough neurological examination, I determine which part of the nervous system is not functioning properly. After twenty years in practice, I have observed that almost all of my migraine patients have a high mesencephalic output. As I have stated earlier, there are three parts of the brainstem: the top, middle, and lower portions. Normally, the brain fires down to the lower brainstem (ponto-medullary), which slows down the upper brainstem (mesencephalon). This is called the neo-cortical-thalamo-hypothalamo-ponto-medullary reticular activating system. In migraine patients, this reticular activating system fails, allowing the mesencephalon to fire at a very high rate.

Activation of the mesencephalon will cause an increase in pulse and heart rate, and the mesencephalic reticular activating system, the area within the mesencephalon that controls sleep patterns, will cause an inability to sleep. The patient may experience increased warmth, increased sweating, and sensitivity to light. This light sensitivity forces migraine sufferers to retreat into a dark room during a migraine. A migraine sufferer is light-sensitive because the pupil fails to constrict, due to a decreased firing of the third cranial nerve. The origin of the third cranial nerve is located in the mesencephalon. Other symptoms associated with a high mesencephalic output may include urinary tract infections. If you recall the discussion from Chapter 5, the mesencephalon stops a person from going to the bathroom. When a patient is unable to completely void the urine, a bacterial infection will result.

In just about every migraine case, I notice a condition in which the eye rotates into the midline when following a pencil toward the nose, then bounces out. This condition is called an exophoria. My personal observation is that with migraine patients, it is usually a 2:1 ratio that the left eye is exophoric as compared to the right.

My purpose as a chiropractic neurologist is to slow the mesencephalon, or upper brainstem. Once I have inhibited, or slowed, the mesencephalic output, the migraine headaches usually disappear.

Jesse
History:

Jesse, a 28 year-old male, had been suffering with migraine headaches for ten years. The headaches were progressively becoming worse, and at the time of presentation, he was experiencing intermittent vomiting. Medical doctors and chiropractors had treated Jesse without success.

Examination:

Upon examination, I observed a left corectasia - a large left pupil. I also found a decrease in muscle tone in the left arm and leg and a decrease in the optokinetic tape testing when moving the tape to the left. Upon moving the optokinetic tape to the patient's left, the parietal lobe slow pursues the eyes to the left, the frontal lobe fast refixates the eyes, or moves the eyes to the right, and the right cerebellum terminates, or stops, the eye movement. Jesse suffered from a decrease in the frequency of firing of his left parietal lobe, left frontal lobe, and right cerebellum. Romberg's sign (standing with his feet together and eyes closed) and Tandem walk (walking heel to toe) revealed a severe global sway, meaning that he swayed back and forth. In many cases, a patient will fall to one side while testing Romberg's sign; this is indicative of a problem with the cerebellum on that side. Rapid hand acceleration, finger to nose, and past pointing were all decreased on his right side. A left palatal paresis was also noted. The soft palate is located on each side of the uvula (the thing that hangs down from the roof of your mouth), and when the patient says "ah," the palate should rise and fall. In Jesse's case, his left soft palate was not rising and falling. The results of all of these tests revealed a high frequency of firing of the mesencephalon.

I chose to manipulate the right side of the Jesse's body to fire the joint receptors, muscle receptors, and tendon receptors up the spinal column to the right cerebellum. These receptors excite large diameter nerves called 1B afferents; these nerves fire into the back part of the spinal column, called the dorsal spinal cerebellar tract, then fire up to the same-side cerebellum. The cerebellum will then fire to the opposite brain. The opposite brain in turn will fire down to the lower brainstem (ponto-medullary), which will slow the upper brainstem (mesencephalon). The lower brainstem will inhibit the mesencephalic output, and the patient's migraines should therefore subside after approximately three to four weeks of treatment. After using these specific treatment modalities with Jesse, he no longer suffers from migraine headaches. Here is what Jesse had to say:

"After 10 Years My Migraines Are Gone"
I suffered from migraine headaches for 10 long years. I would experience blurry vision before a migraine and over time the headaches were becoming worse. Movement aggravated my condition. While sleep and Excedrin Migraine provided some relief. I went to Apple Medical Clinic for help. The doctors diagnosed my condition and finally after 10 years my migraines are gone!

Alice
History:
Alice, a 50 year-old female, had been suffering from migraine

headaches for forty years. She stated that her migraine headaches began when she was nine or ten years old. She would suffer migraine headaches at least three to four times per week. Again, numerous medical doctors, chiropractors, and physical therapists had treated Alice without success. She stated that she had been treating with one chiropractor for over two years with little results. Alice had tried a multitude of medications without relief.

Examination:

Upon examination, I found many symptoms similar to those of other migraine patients. I observed a severe right exophoria (the right eye will pop out upon moving the pen toward the nose), a right corectasia (a large right pupil), and a decreased pupillary response on the left (when shining light into the left eye, instead of constricting and holding, the pupil got bigger immediately). I also observed a decrease in optokinetic tape testing when moving the tape to the right. I began a treatment protocol of adjusting Alice with an activator (a small hand-held instrument) on the left side. Alice is like many of the migraine patients that I have treated; they cannot tolerate a structural adjustment (popping and cracking) on the neck. Alice also received a warm caloric on the left side. A warm caloric will increase the flow of endolymph, a gelatinous material in the semicircular canals of the ear. The endolymph stimulates hair cells in those canals that in turn excite the vestibular nerve, which will increase the frequency of firing of the same-side, or left, cerebellum. The left cerebellum will fire to the right side of the brain, which will fire to the lower brainstem (ponto-medullary) and slow the upper brainstem (mesencephalon). Upon utilizing these treatment modalities, the patient progressively improved. She is currently under care, and she states that her migraines are less frequent and much less intense. When she initiated care, her headache pain intensity - on a scale where "0" is no pain and "10" is severe pain - was rated at a "10." Her headache intensity is now rated at a "2" and all of her objective findings improved.

Ginny
History:

Ginny, a 68 year-old female, had been suffering from migraine headaches for years. When she presented to my office, she had been under the care of various medical doctors, and at the time of her presentation, she was under the care of another chiropractor. When she entered our office, she assumed that she was seeing another medical doctor. When I explained to her that I was a chiropractic neurologist, she became very upset, especially since it was a one-hour drive from her home. She stated that she already had a chiropractor and did not need to see anyone else. I said that I was different and that as a chiropractic neurologist, I have additional training and use different treatment modalities than the general chiropractor. She agreed to come back for a second visit to view her x-rays. She stated that her headaches were on the right side, and although the headaches were constant, they would vary in intensity.

I adjusted Ginny on the right side to increase the firing, or impulses, to the right cerebellum and left-brain. She also received auditory stimulation consisting of ocean sounds in the right ear for 5-10 minutes. Over the course of the next few treatments, her sleeping improved to eight to nine hours straight through; previously, she would get up several times during a night with headaches. As her treatment progressed, her symptoms steadily decreased. After a few visits, I incorporated olfactory stimulation. Olfactory stimulation consists of smelling different scents; this action fires directly into the temporal lobe of the brain. Your sight, touch, taste, and hearing all go through a relay station called the thalamus, a walnut sized area in the brain. The thalamus then fires to the cortex, or brain. Smell, however, goes directly to the brain - specifically, the temporal lobe. Ginny even found that when she woke up with a headache one morning and did the olfactory stimulation at home, her headache disappeared. At the end of her treatment trial, Ginny was headache-free. She said that she and her husband would be spending the winter in Arizona, and if she required my services again, she would certainly call me.

Jean
History:

Jean, a 56 year-old married female, presented to my office in March of 2000 complaining of headaches radiating down to the right side of her neck. She stated that her headaches began approximately three to four years before. Numerous medical doctors had treated her for her condition, and she was prescribed many different medications with little success. She found that over-the-counter medications such as Advil were just as effective as her prescription medications. She had also been under physical therapy, and she stated that her neck exercises did provide some relief. Her pain varied from morning to afternoon, and her severe headaches would occur 1-2 times per month and last anywhere from 3-5 days.

Examination:

Upon examining Jean, I found weakness in muscle strength in the right side, a right exophoria, a right palatal paresis, and a decrease in the right optokinetic tape testing for the parietal lobe, right frontal lobe and left cerebellum. When testing Romberg's sign and Tandem walk, Jean exhibited a moderate sway. Rapid acceleration of the hands and finger to nose were also decreased on the left, indicative of a decreased left cerebellar function and decreased right cortical frequency of firing (impulses).

I treated Jean with unilateral manipulations, or adjustments, on her left side to increase the frequency of firing of the left cerebellum and right-brain. Jean received T.E.N.S. (Transelectrical nerve stimulation) at a subthreshold level (meaning she could not feel it) on the arm and cervical spine to increase the frequency of firing of the left cerebellum. I also used heat on Jean's cervical spine to increase the cerebellar frequency of firing.

Two treatment modalities that worked very well for Jean were visual and auditory stimulation. Auditory stimulation - ocean sounds in the left ear - increases the frequency of firing of the opposite temporal lobe via the mesencephalon. Visual stimulation on the left side crosses through the mesencephalon and increases impulses in the right-brain. Both visual and auditory stimulation are monitored by blood pressure, pulse rate, tissue saturation of oxygen, and other neurological tests.

Jean stated that my examination was one of the most thorough examinations she had ever received, including the exams from many of her previous medical doctors. After three to four weeks of treatments, we noticed an improvement with her headaches. After two to three months, Jean was headache-free. I released Jean to a PRN status, meaning that she could return as needed. I do this with many of my patients - I leave the decision up to them. Some patients continue to check in a few times per year just to see how things are going in their bodies, and others move on to a PRN status. I treat patients the way I would like to be treated. The key is to give patients an option.

About a year later, Jean was on vacation in Canada and began to experience dizziness. The vertigo progressively became worse, and when Jean returned to Appleton, her medical doctor prescribed the medication Meclizine. Much to her dismay, the Meclizine made her dizziness worse. While she was in my office for her check-up, she mentioned that she had some problems with vertigo, and she asked if I could help her. I said, "Certainly, vertigo is one of the cases with which I have a lot of success." I performed another examination on Jean, and interestingly enough, our findings were exactly opposite of those in the first examination. This is why a doctor should never treat the patient exactly the same way every time the patient presents to his office. The body is dynamic and is constantly changing, as Jean's case shows. After we had treated Jean for about 4-6 weeks, her dizziness was gone. Jean continues to see me on a maintenance schedule once every 8-12 weeks.

Sandy
History:

This 40 year-old female presented to my office complaining of constant headaches after being involved in a car accident. During the summer of 2001, Sandy's automobile was struck from behind while the driver was talking on his cell phone. At the time of the accident, Sandy was looking to her right and was not able to brace herself for impact. Studies have shown that there are a significant number of injuries related to soft tissue (muscles, tendons, and ligaments), although the insurance industry denies it. The most recent studies have found that when hit from behind at only 8 mph, your car receives 2 ½ G's of force, your shoulder strap receives 4 G's of force, and your head and neck receive 5 G's of force. Even in a low impact collision, the transfer of energy to the head and neck is twice the energy transferred to the car. Occupants are subject to much more force in low-impact collisions where the vehicle is not damaged than in more severe collisions where the vehicle plastically deforms. Recently, I was watching a NASCAR race, and a car involved in a collision was blown to pieces, yet the driver got up and walked away. The impact or load is expressed in the dynamic break-up of the automobile. When there is no dynamic break-up of the automobile, the occupant suffers the most injury. When a 3,500 lb. car strikes the rear-end of another car, it may transmit a force of up to 25 tons. The amount of damage that an automobile receives may bear little relationship to the patient's injury. Insurance companies are aware of all of this. As a result, they have implemented a computer formula that makes it extremely difficult for occupants of a low-impact collision to make any type of claim, based on the insurance company's "evidence." The insurance companies "are your neighbor" and "keep you in good hands" if you are one of their clients. God forbid if you are one of the occupants that one of their clients has hit. You are anything but a "good friend" or "neighbor." The last thing the insurance company wants is a claim against their company.

Sandy had been treating with three different medical doctors and chiropractors at the time of presentation. She stated that she was having trouble sleeping, was suffering from headaches, and was experiencing neck pain that radiated down into her arms. Sandy exhibited muscle weakness on the left side, a severe muscle spasm throughout the cervical and thoracic spine, a decrease in olfactory perception on the left, and a decrease in the optokinetic tape testing. She also exhibited a left exophoria upon convergence, a left palatal paresis, a moderate sway when testing Romberg's sign and Tandem walk, and numerous positive orthopedic tests. Over the course of her first eighteen-visit treatment trial, Sandy responded quite favorably.

Susan
History:

Susan, a 35 year-old female, had been suffering with migraines since the age of twelve. In the five years prior to presentation, Susan stated that her migraine headaches occurred daily, whereas previously they had only been occurring one to two times per week. Susan suffered from classical migraines in that she experienced visual disturbances. After a visual disturbance, she would experience a sharp, intense pain in the front part of her skull that radiated to the back. She also stated that she had trouble with her jaw, known as TMJ. This is specifically common in migraine headache sufferers because the TMJ center is located in the mesencephalon.

Because of her high mesencephalic frequency of firing, Susan was extremely light-sensitive. She also experienced cervical spine pain that radiated into the shoulders, and she suffered from cramping and irregularity during her menstrual cycle. She noted that the headaches became more intense during her menstrual period. She also stated that any activities, smells, changes in weather, and stress would make her migraines worse. As of late, she had become more irritable, depressed, and fatigued because she had been unable to find a doctor to resolve her condition. Because of her headaches, depression, and fatigue, she had been unable to work or participate in any outside activities. It was to the point where Susan sat in her room and stared at the wall for the majority of the day.

She stated that the pain had been so severe that she tried every type of therapy that one can imagine. She had been under the care of an abundance of medical doctors and chiropractors, without results. She had treated with two dentists who prescribed splints to treat the migraines, but the splints made the migraines worse. She also tried acupuncture, biofeedback therapy, visual imagery, physical therapy, and occupational therapy. She had been on a number of medications that either had no effect or made the migraines worse. At the time of presentation, Susan was on Oxycodone, Excedrin, and Ibuprofen. She had been on a number of seizure medications in the past, including Topamax, Neurontin, and Imitrex, without results. She had been under the care of medical doctors at the Mayo Clinic in Rochester, Minnesota, the Marshfield Clinic in Marshfield, Wisconsin, and the Diamond Headache Clinic in Chicago, Illinois. Doctors were accusing Susan of being lazy, just imagining the headaches so she would not have to work. This was not the case.

Susan was also being treated for rebound headaches, meaning that Tylenol or other pain relievers were causing what they were meant to cure. In Susan, these pain pills had thrown her body's natural pain-control system out of whack, causing the headaches to return after the medication wore off. She already had gone through detoxification in the hospital for rebound headaches, and her neurologist was proposing another treatment regime of detoxification to remove all of her medications.

Upon filling out her case history form, Susan stated that she tries to stay positive and prays that eventually something will help her to get on with her life.

Examination:

Upon examination, I found a severe left corectasia (the pupil was extremely large). This is a result of the third cranial nerve failing to constrict the pupil. A severe left exophoria, a severe decrease in the left optokinetic tape testing, a severe blepherospasm, and a left palatal paresis were also present. When standing with her feet together and eyes closed (Romberg's Sign), Susan would fall to her left. These neurological signs indicate the decreased function of the brainstem and cerebellum. There is no way that a patient can "fake" a large pupil, exophoria, or palatal paresis. One could say that she could fake falling to her left, but when a patient does not know what the doctor is looking for, it is hard to fake it.

I began treating Susan with light extremity adjustments. No structural adjustments (popping and cracking) were made to Susan's spine because this type of treatment could overstimulate metabolic capacity and make her headaches worse. I also tested Susan neurologically for a number of food allergies and found that she was allergic to eggs, dairy, and sugar. After clearing out the food allergies, performing an intensive regime of light adjustments on the right side of her body, and eventually administering auditory stimulation, Susan's pain intensity began to decrease. She had initially presented with a daily pain intensity of "7," but by the sixth week of treatments, Susan was experiencing a pain intensity of "3." At the end of twelve weeks, Susan's pain was down to a "1," and on some days, Susan was headache-free. At this point Susan's husband received a job offer in California, so I referred her to a chiropractic neurologist. Susan has family in the Wisconsin area, enabling her to return a few times per year, and she asked if I could still treat her. I told her that I would be happy to. Susan was extremely grateful, and she has referred a number of friends to our office.

Christopher

History:

This 15 year-old male presented to our office suffering from migraine headaches since age three. Christopher's mother stated that he also suffered from light sensitivity and blurred vision. His pediatrician had numerous tests and studies performed which were all negative. Christopher's headaches would radiate from the back of his head to the middle of his forehead, and he experienced severe cervical spine pain that radiated down into his shoulders. His headaches were becoming so severe that they interfered with his daily activities and sports, and Christopher was an avid basketball and baseball player.

Examination:

Christopher exhibited a decreased left optokinetic tape test, a left corectasia, a hypermetria up to the right and down to the left, and a moderate sway upon testing Romberg's sign (standing feet together and eyes closed). His treatment regime included structural adjustments to the right side of his body to increase function of the right cerebellum and left-brain. Christopher received electrical stimulation on his right arm, and he received heat therapy to increase the frequency of firing of the muscle, joint, and tendon receptors that fire up to the right cerebellum. We also treated Christopher with a warm caloric in the right ear to stimulate the endolymph in the semi-circular canals, which in turn will increase the frequency of firing to the vestibular nerve by exciting the hair canals.

I am happy to report that Christopher responded to care almost immediately. At the end of his twelve-week treatment trial, Christopher was completely free of headaches. At that time, I put Christopher on a maintenance schedule to see him one time per month. I do not anticipate a return of the migraine headaches due to massive improvement in his objective findings (especially the left corectasia and hypermetria).

(Please note that the preceding case histories are only a few of the thousands of patients that we have helped in our clinic in the past 20 years.)

Chapter 8:
Fibromyalgia

*"God may forgive your sins,
but your nervous system won't."*
-Alfred Korzybski: *Healthways*

Fibromyalgia is a form of generalized muscular pain and fatigue that affects almost 5 million Americans. It is estimated that as many as 10-15 million more individuals go undiagnosed. The term *fibromyalgia* means pain in the muscles and connective tissue surrounding the muscles, ligaments, and tendons. Many medical doctors insist that a patient must have a certain number (11 out of 18) of positive trigger points (painful areas) in order to be diagnosed with fibromyalgia. Presently, there are some medical doctors who feel that there is no need to find any positive trigger points in order to diagnose a patient with fibromyalgia. My feeling is "who cares?" Fibromyalgia is a name, a label so to speak. "Here you go Mrs. Jones, let's put you in this neat little fibromyalgia box so we can treat you with medication, exercise, and stretching." Fibromyalgia to me, literally means, "I have pain all over and I'm really tired." Fibromyalgia cannot be revealed by an abnormal lab finding; the diagnosis instead depends mostly on a person's report, complaints, and feelings. Pain is the most prominent symptom of fibromyalgia, and it generally occurs through the entire body, although it may start in one region, such as the neck and shoulders, and spread to other areas over a period of time.

The majority of patients with fibromyalgia experience moderate to severe fatigue. The patient may experience lack of energy, decreased exercise endurance, and the kind of exhaustion that results from the flu or lack of sleep. At times, the fatigue is more of a problem than the pain. Abdominal pain, bloating, alternating constipation and diarrhea, migraine headaches, and muscular tension headaches are all part of the fibromyalgia syndrome. Some patients may suffer from a frequency of urination. The skin and circulation can be sensitive to temperature changes, resulting in a temporary - or sometimes permanent - change in skin color. Patients may suffer from a mental fatigue in which they feel they are literally in some type of "brain fog."

In treating fibromyalgia patients over the years, I have found that many (not all) fibromyalgia patients have been under some type of severe stress in their lives. Many fibromyalgia patients have suffered sexual abuse, verbal abuse, emotional abuse, financial stress, or all of the above. Keep in mind that this is simply my clinical observation.

Fibromyalgia patients, as well as all other chronic pain patients (symptoms lasting longer than six months), must be monitored closely. Before and after treatment, blood pressure, pulse, and tissue saturation of oxygen should be taken, and positive neurological tests should be monitored. If the patient is not closely monitored, it is possible to overstimulate a patient's metabolic capacity and increase the severity of the symptoms.

In every case of fibromyalgia that I have treated over the past six years, I have found a high mesencephalic output. Remember the brainstem? It consists of the mesencephalon (top portion), pons (middle), and medulla (lower). High output in the mesencephalon causes the symptoms that fibromyalgia patients experience. Sensitivity to light, increased warmth or sweating, inability to sleep, increased pulse or heart rate, urinary tract infections, pain, and fatigue are all classic signs that the mesencephalon (upper brainstem) is overfiring as a result of the ponto-medullary (lower brainstem) region failing to inhibit it, or slow it down.

Light sensitivity is one result of a high mesencephalic output. The third and fourth cranial nerves are based in the mesencephalon, and the third cranial nerve allows the pupil to constrict. When the third cranial nerve is not firing properly, the pupil will dilate and the patient will become sensitive to light.

A patient's inability to sleep is a result of an overfiring of the mesencephalic reticular activating system (figure 8-1), the area in the mesencephalon that controls sleep patterns. When it is firing at a very high rate, you are awake, and when it is firing at a very low

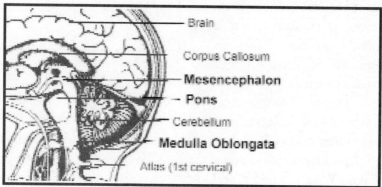

Figure 8-1

rate, you are asleep. The mesencephalic reticular activating system is firing at its greatest rate at approximately 3:00 p.m. and at its lowest at approximately 3:00 a.m. Chronic fatigue usually accompanies fibromyalgia due to the abnormal firing of the mesencephalic reticular activating system.

The mesencephalon excites an area in the spinal cord - called the intermedial lateral cell nucleus, or IML (figure 8-2) - that fires down to the SA and AV nodes, the electrical areas of the heart. The SA node, located on the right side of the heart, and the AV node, located on the left side of the heart, act like circuit breakers that control the electrical impulses which control the heart rate. When the ponto-medullary region fails to inhibit the mesencephalon, the IML fails to function. This will cause abnormal firing of the SA and AV nodes, which in turn will cause heart palpitations or a change in heart rate. Generally, a patient with a decreased firing of the right brain will suffer from tachycardia, or an increased heart rate, and a person with a decreased firing of the left brain will suffer from arrhythmia, or an irregular heart rate.

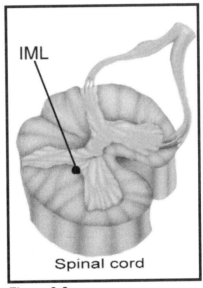

Figure 8-2

Pain is the final symptom that results from a high mesencephalic output. The mesencephalon drives the IML, and when the IML fires down the spinal cord, it causes the adrenal medulla to release norepinephrine and catecholamines into the bloodstream. When these chemicals are released into the bloodstream, they stimulate pain fibers, called type-C or nociceptive fibers. This is the reason why a fibromyalgia patient feels pain all over; he/she feels pain in the left leg one day, pain in the right shoulder the next, and mid-back pain with a headache on the third.

Symptoms Usually Associated with a High (abnormal) Firing of the Mesencephalon

Light sensitivity
Inability to Sleep
Increased or Irregular Heartbeat
Increased Sweating (warmth)
Pain

Darlene
History:

Darlene, a 50 year-old female, had been suffering from fibromyalgia for over seven years. She had been dealing with over-all pain and worsening fatigue for several years. When she arose in the morning, she was hardly able to move. She stated that she would have to force herself to go to work. By early afternoon, her pain and headaches were unbearable, and her condition forced her to curtail her time at work. By early evening, she was completely exhausted and was forced to drop out of many of her social activities. Her suffering was also adversely affecting her marriage. Numerous medical doctors, chiropractors, and physical therapists had treated Darlene. She had undergone a variety of tests, which included a complete blood work-up, an MRI, a CT scan, and an EMG. She had also been on special nutritional diets that required her to eliminate specific foods in order to alleviate some of her pain. She had been on a low dose of antibiotics, and she had tried many different types of medications. Her condition continually worsened. Another chiropractor had treated her for many years, and she stated that his treatments would provide her with short periods of relief. The chronic pain stemmed from the neck, or cervical spine, and radiated into the shoulder and down into her arms. Her lower back pain would radiate down into her legs. When under severe stress, she would experience severe migraine headaches. All of these symptoms left her unable to sleep, which resulted in a sharp drop in her energy level.

Examination:

Upon examination of Darlene (see Chapter 4: Examination), I observed a severe right exophoria (the right eye bounces out when you move the pen toward the eyes) and a decrease in optokinetic tape testing to the right. Normally, when you move the optokinetic tape to a patient's right (figure 8-3), the parietal lobe of the brain (figure 8-4) picks up the slow pursuit to the right. The slow pursuit is approximately 50 degrees per second (pinhead time again). The frontal lobe (front part of the brain) refixates the eyes back to the left at approximately 300 to 700 degrees per second, and the left cerebellum will terminate, or stop, the eye movement. Darlene exhibited a decrease in all aspects of the optokinetic tape testing. I also observed a severe blepherospasm. Blepherospasm is a big, fancy word meaning that when you close your eyes, your eyelids

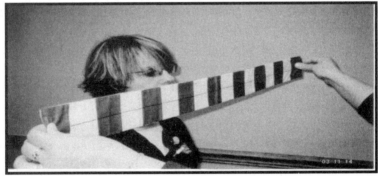

Figure 8-3

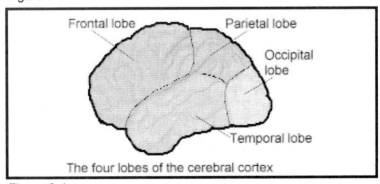

Figure 8-4

twitch like crazy. The eyelids are under control of the third cranial nerve, which has its origin in the upper brainstem, or mesencephalon. Darlene also exhibited a decrease in smell on her right side. Taste, touch, sound, and sight all go through the walnut-shaped area of the brain called the thalamus. The thalamus will then send impulses to the cortex, or brain. Your smell (olfactory)-(figure 8-5), however, goes directly to the temporal lobe, not through the relay station, the thalamus. Olfactory stimulation is a very powerful treatment modality because of the direct connection to the brain. A right corectasia (large right pupil) (figure 8-6) was also observed. A large right pupil is caused by the third cranial nerve not functioning properly. I also observed a palatal paresis on the right. A palatal paresis is noted by having the patient say "ah"

a number of times, then observing if the palate near the back of the mouth rises and falls. The uvula, or "thing that hangs down in the back of your mouth," is not involved. The palate is under the control of the ninth and tenth cranial nerves, whose origin is in the lower brainstem.

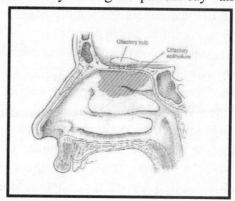

Figure 8-5

Darlene exhibited a moderate sway upon testing the Romberg's

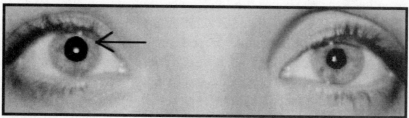

Figure 8-6

sign (standing with feet together and eyes closed) and Tandem walk (walking heel to toe). All orthopedic tests were positive in the cervical and lumbar spine. I found a decrease in the range of motion in the cervical (neck) and lumbar (lower back) spine, along with pain throughout all ranges of motion.

I thought Darlene could handle a structural (popping and cracking) manipulation because of her exam findings. In many cases of fibromyalgia, patients cannot handle structural manipulation because the high level of stimulation will aggravate symptoms. Along with manipulation, we used electrical stimulation and moist heat on the left side to increase the firing, or impulses, of the left cerebellum. We also used cervical traction. Cervical traction promotes a slow stretch of the muscle which fires a different pathway up to the cerebellum. Finally, we used auditory and visual stimulation. Auditory and visual stimulation will enter the upper brainstem (mesencephalon) and increase impulses to the opposite brain. In many cases, we will use auditory stimulation on the side opposite of decreased brain function. In Darlene's case, this was her left side. We may use ocean sounds, Mozart, or other nature sounds, depending on the amount of stimulation needed. Visual stimulation can be performed with a number of treatment modalities, one of which is viewing faces. The viewing of faces stimulates the amygdala, located deep in the temporal lobe. Viewing familiar faces will stimulate the left amygdala, while viewing unfamiliar faces will stimulate the right. Looking at large letters made up of small letters also increases impulses to the cerebellum. If you look at the large letters, you excite the left cerebellum, which fires up to the right brain. If you look at the small letters that make up the large letters, you excite the right cerebellum, which fires up to the left brain. In another form of visual stimulation, the patient views moving colored blocks on a screen. In Darlene's case, I used the block therapy, and she responded extremely well.

After approximately eight weeks of care, Darlene experienced remarkable improvement. Her energy level had greatly improved, and the heavy fatigue had lifted. On very busy days, she would not get "bone tired" by the evening. Her sleep patterns had greatly improved, and she was in much less pain. She stated that her restless leg syndrome occurred only occasionally, not nightly. The leg, foot, hip, and back pain, along with the neck and shoulder pain, has improved to the point where she is hardly aware of any pain at all. Previously, Darlene would experience chest pain when walking long distances, but after her treatments, she no longer experiences pain.

Due to the severity of her condition, I continue to treat Darlene 4-6 times per year. When people say, "Once you go to a chiropractor, you always have to go," I respond, "You're right!" Once you go to a dentist, you always have to go. You see a dentist twice a year, so why shouldn't you see a chiropractor a few times per year to have your nervous system checked? This is especially important if you have suffered from a chronic health condition. Here's what Darlene had to say:

April 8, 2002
Dear Sirs,

I understand there is some question of why Dr. Johnson is different from other chiropractors. Let me share my experience.

I have been dealing with overall pain and a worsening fatigue for several years. One-and-a-half years ago I became chronically fatigued. I rose in the morning hardly able to move. I had to force myself to go to work. By early afternoon, my headaches were unbearable. I had to cut back on my work days. By evening, I was totally spent. Had to drop out of many activities. It affected my marriage because I had nothing left for my husband. He was also doing most of the housework and a lot of meal preparation. I was losing control of my life. I had sought help for many years. My allergist tried different treatments to help with the pain, fatigue, and headaches. He took special blood tests for arthritis. Tests for several years in a row checking my adrenal system. Put me on special nutritional diets - eliminating certain foods. Had me on a low-dose antibiotic to help control the pain. He tried other medica-

tions, but everything continued to get worse, and I also went to my regular doctor with my complaints. For a while he put me on one medication and then another. Finally, he sent me to a specialist to thoroughly check out my adrenal system. Found no problem. I had blood tests for arthritis - came back negative. He ordered an MRI of my brain - negative. I had a bone density test - fine for my age. Cholesterol a little high but I brought it down with diet. Had an ultrasound to recheck an old cyst on my ovary - all well. All in all, they found no apparent cause for all my pain, fatigue and severe headaches, and it becomes very discouraging when no doctors can help. In the few minutes you get in their offices, it is hard to make them believe it's not all in your head.

I also had been going to another chiropractor for many years. He helped some for short periods of time. I had a chronic problem with my upper back and neck, especially a very painful trigger point on the top right shoulder between my neck and shoulder blade. It would be so hard and painful that I would drop objects when lifting them. This chiropractor worked on the knowledge of muscles - it would help some temporarily, but it always came back. This pain would spread to my head and set off severe headaches.

Since I've been under Dr. Johnson's care I have made much improvement. My fatigue is mostly gone, and I'm sleeping sound again. My energy level is way up. My headaches are now very few and mild. Also, the doctor and his therapist have gotten rid of that painful trigger point. I'm totally rid of it. Dr. Johnson also has taught me several things I can do at home to help with pain control. I still have my fibromyalgia, but now I go through my days mostly pain-free. My need to see Dr. Johnson is growing less and less.

Dr. Johnson has helped me regain my life and it was done without drugs. All the other doctors failed to find the fibromyalgia or treat it. People who are very sick and have exhausted their search with other doctors - come to Dr. Johnson and get help. I'm so thankful I found Dr. Johnson.

Sincerely,
Darlene

Christie
History:

This 25 year-old female presented to Apple Medical Clinic for evaluation and treatment of headaches, neck pain, and lower back pain. Christie began to suffer from these symptoms after an auto accident. She had not yet been diagnosed with fibromyalgia, but chronic fatigue did accompany her condition. She also had numerous tender points indicative of fibromyalgia, and she has a family history of fibromyalgia. Both her mother and aunt have been diagnosed with fibromyalgia, and I informed Christie that she could also be suffering from the disease. She had been under the care of numerous medical doctors and chiropractors with few results. Christie stated that the pain in her neck started at the back of her head and radiated up into the frontal aspect of the skull and down into the neck and shoulder area. She also experienced an occasional stabbing pain in her mid-back area, and her lower back pain would become worse with daily activities such as sitting, bending, or lying down.

Christie also related that she had difficulty sleeping, heart palpitations, light sensitivity, and frequent urinary tract infections. The causes of the first three symptoms are discussed in the previous section, and urinary tract infections, like the other symptoms, are caused by a high frequency of firing of the mesencephalon. The mesencephalon restricts urinary output when it is overfiring, causing a stasis of urine. This contributes to urinary tract infections because of the high bacteria content of static urine.

Examination:

Upon examination of Christie, I observed a severe blepherospasm, an indication of a decrease in brain function. A blepherospasm, a focal dystonia, occurs when the eyelids twitch uncontrollably after the patient closes her eyes. Christie also showed a decrease in brain function in the optokinetic tape test. Upon moving the optokinetic tape to the patient's left side, the left part of the brain, specifically the parietal lobe, picks up a slow pursuit to the left. The left frontal lobe of the brain will quickly refixate the eyes back to the right, and the opposite (right) cerebellum will terminate the eye movement. All of these functions were decreased in Christie's case. When standing with her feet together and eyes closed (Romberg's Sign), Christie fell back and to her right, which is an indication of a decrease in the cerebellar frequency of firing, or impulses. I also observed a decrease in the rapid hand acceleration on the right side. When touching her right index finger to her nose, she would completely miss her nose.

After a comprehensive examination and specific x-rays, I found that Christie had lost the normal cervical curve. The cerebellum controls the spinal musculature, and in Christie's case, the cerebellum was not functioning. The spinal musculature therefore spasm, and Christie lost the lordotic, or forward, curve in her cervical spine or neck.

Christie's initial treatments were unilateral manipulations on the right side to increase the frequency of firing of muscle, joint, and tendon receptors. These receptors will then increase the firing to the same-side (right) cerebellum. T.E.N.S. (trans-electrical nerve stimulation) and ultrasound treatments were utilized to stimulate neurons involved in the musculature to also increase the frequency of firing. Heat therapy was used to increase the metabolic and healing rate of the involved tissues, and a warm caloric of water was administered into the right ear to stimulate the same-side cerebellum. Warm water increases the frequency of firing of the same-side semicircular canals, small canals inside of the ears. A gelatinous material called endolymph lies inside these canals. When Jell-O is heated, it becomes liquefied, and the same concept occurs inside of the ear. When the endolymph is heated, it liquifies, and an increase in the movement of endolymph causes an increased stimulation of the hair cells inside of the canals. This stimulation fires the vestibular nerve back to the cerebellum, increasing the frequency of firing to the cerebellum. As with all chronic pain patients, oxygen was administered via mask per order from our medical doctor, increasing the mitochondrial stores of the supporting musculature. Mitochondria are the powerhouses in the muscle cells, and an increase in the mitochondrial stores aids rehabilitation and increases fuel delivery to the nervous system.

After Christie's six-week initial treatment period of three treatments per week, we found remarkable progress both subjectively (symptoms) and objectively (testing). As a result, we decreased Christie's treatment protocol to one treatment per week. We are currently seeing Christie on a weekly basis, and she continues to make exceptional progress.

Linda
History:

Linda, a 50 year-old female, presented to my office in February of 2002. She had been diagnosed with fibromyalgia by a rheumatologist and stated that she had suffered from this condition since 1986. Any type of bending or sitting would aggravate her condition. She had been to several chiropractors, medical doctors, and physical therapists only to hear such responses as "learn to live with the pain," "it's all in your head," or "I can't help you." This was a very frustrating and hopeless time in her life. Linda related that she would dread having to wake up in the morning. The knowledge of the severe pain that she would have to endure that day was becoming too much to bear. She stated that it sometimes hurt to walk only a few steps, to raise her arms, or to sit or stand for any period of time. If someone touched her arm or hand in a friendly gesture, the pain would shoot through her entire body. She was unable to get adequate rest and sleep. Her concentration level was very low. Although she was trying to keep a positive attitude, it seemed that she would only receive negative responses from the medical field.

Examination:

Upon examination, Linda exhibited a severe left exophoria and a severe sway when standing with her feet together and eyes closed (also known as the Romberg's position). A palatal paresis and a decrease in olfactory perception on the left side were also noted. Overall, just about every test I performed on Linda was positive. When she initially presented to our office, she stated that her pain level was a "10." After approximately three months, Linda stated that her pain level was at a "4" on a scale where "0" is no pain and "10" is severe pain. Upon initial presentation, she was taking up to five different medications a day. By the time she dismissed herself from care at a pain level of "2," she was only taking an occasional Extra-Strength Tylenol. She was astonished that after all these years of suffering, she finally found someone to listen to her and care for her whole body, not just the isolated medical dilemma she was going through. Unfortunately, Linda was in an HMO, which meant that she was paying for the care out of her own pocket. As a patient in our office, however, she eliminated expensive testing and prescription medications, and she was looking at long term results, thereby saving her insurance company money. Linda was kind enough to write a testimonial that I have enclosed. I find it very gratifying to help patients such as Linda.

May 10, 2002
To Whom It May Concern:

Back in 1986, I was diagnosed with fibromyalgia. Ten years prior to this, I had the same symptoms, spending a lot of time and money going to several chiropractors, M.D.'s, and therapists, only to hear such responses as, "learn to live with the pain," "it's all in your head," or "I can't help you." This was a very frustrating and hopeless time in my life. I dreaded having to wake up in the morning to start my day, knowing the pain I would have to endure. There were times when it hurt to walk a few steps, to raise my arms, or to sit or stand for any period of time, and if someone would touch my arm or hand in a friendly gesture, the pain shot through my whole body. I was not getting adequate sleep and rest, my concentration level was at its lowest, and it was hard to keep a positive attitude when all you hear is negative responses from the medical field.

I have been under Dr. Johnson's care for just shy of three months. I came in with a pain level that was way over a "10," I am now at a "4," only to get better! I was taking up to five different medications a day, and now I only take an occasional Extra-Strength Tylenol, if needed. I was astonished and bewildered that after all these years of so much pain, I finally had hope and someone to listen to me and care for my whole being, not just the isolated medical dilemma I was going through. I never thought it possible that I could live in a pain-free world. I'm not there yet, but with Dr. Johnson's help, I know it's in the near future.

Insurance companies these days are so concerned with cost savings and cutting corners, and yet they don't take that time to look at alternative medicine as a means to an end. They need to look at the whole picture and ask themselves, in the long run, who comes out the winner? As a patient of Dr. Johnson, I am eliminating expensive testing and prescribed medications. I am looking at long-term and permanent results, also saving my insurance company money on unnecessary tests and medications that would have been prescribed by M.D.'s. It might cost more up front, but in the long run, there is a cost savings regarding repeated office visits, refilling prescriptions, and going through expensive and repeated tests.

When I'm the patient, I like to see some genuine concern and effort on the part of a doctor and that is what I get when I see Dr. Johnson. He does everything he can possibly do for permanent results, not a temporary fix. Dr. Johnson is concerned with your whole being and is very informational with his procedures. When you leave his office, you feel you are getting positive results and seeing improvement, and I never dreamed this was possible.

I wished I had known about Dr. Johnson and his treatment years ago. It would have saved me a lot of pain and sleepless nights, not to mention the money that was spent. Until you have walked in the shoes of someone with fibromyalgia, you have no idea what it is like!

A VERY SATISFIED PATIENT OF DR. JOHNSON!

Linda

Diane

History:

Diane, a 59 year-old female, presented to my office complaining of severe pain and numbness over her entire body that had affected her for many years. She had been diagnosed with fibromyalgia a number of years before by a rheumatologist, and she had been under the care of many chiropractors and medical doctors. She had multiple imaging studies and nerve tests done, all of which were essentially negative. She complained of severe pain in the sacro-illiac region (above the tail bone). Sharp pain radiated down her right leg into her right ankle, and neck pain radiated down into her arms. She stated that going up and down stairs bothered her and that her condition was gradually becoming worse each day. She also suffered from cramping in her legs, numbness in her arms, sleeplessness, loss of balance, and sensitivity to light.

Examination:

Just about every neurological and orthopedic test that I performed on Diane was positive. She exhibited a decreased olfactory perception on the left, a decreased optokinetic tape test on the left, a corectasia on the left, and a left exophoria upon convergence. Her V/A ratio was high on the left, along with a marked palatal paresis. When standing with her feet together and eyes closed, she exhibited a severe global sway. A decrease in the right rapid hand acceleration was observed.

At approximately the fourth or fifth visit, Diane stated that her pain was slightly decreased and she was sleeping much better. Over the course of the next three or four months, Diane's condition continued to greatly improve to the point where she was completely free of pain. She stated that her improvement had been "tremendous!" Upon initial presentation, she was unable to walk up stairs without pain and was only able to take one step at a time. Now, she has no difficulty walking up stairs, and her overall pain and discomfort has disappeared. She has more energy and a better general feeling of well-being then she has had in the past five years. She is able to walk without a limp and is much steadier on her feet. Her balance has greatly improved, and on top of all of this, Diane was able to lose fifty pounds as a direct result of seeing our medical doctor, Dr. Manellema Fernando, a board-certified bariatric physician and specialist in obesity. Dr. Fernando was able to help Diane lose the weight without bariatric surgery, as she does with many of our patients. You can locate a bariatric physician in your area at www.asbp.org. Listen to what Diane had to say:

"My Pain is Gone!"

I had suffered from fibromyalgia for years. I had pain all over, especially in my lower back and hips. I also had suffered from leg cramps, numbness in my arms and legs, sleeplessness, loss of balance, fatigue, and sensitivity to light.

I had numerous tests done, including an EMG and an MRI. The MRI showed a slight disc bulging in the lower back.

I saw the ad for Apple Medical Clinic and decided to give them a try. My improvement has been tremendous! Before my treatment, I could never walk up stairs without pain, and I could only take one step at a time. Now, I have no difficulty walking up stairs. My overall pain and discomfort is now gone. I have more energy and a general feeling of well-being than I have in the past 5 years. I walk without a limp. I am steadier on my feet and do not feel like I will fall. My balance has greatly improved. I feel great!

-Diane

Paula Jean
History:

Paula Jean, a 44 year-old-female, presented to our office complaining of multiple pain syndromes. She suffered from pain in her neck, and she was often plagued by paresthesia, or numbness, in her arms, hands, and fingers. She suffered from migraine headaches and experienced mid-back pain just below the shoulder blade. Her hips were giving her a lot of problems, and she suffered from leg pain and swollen ankles. In addition, she suffered from a severe left-handed tremor. She was continuously waking up during the night, suffered from a severe sensitivity to light, noticed that she would sweat a lot, and experienced an increase in her heart rate. She noticed that in the last two or three years, she had difficulty expressing what she wanted to say. Along with her poor memory, she had experienced episodes of depression and anxiety for some time. She had been taking Bldeprlyl, a drug for tremors, and an inhaler for her asthma.

Examination:

Upon examining Paula Jean, I found that she had lost vibratory sensation and muscle strength in her left side. I observed a right exophoria upon accommodation, a decrease in the right optokinetic tape test, a palatal paresis on the right, and a decrease in the right olfactory perception. Paula Jean also exhibited a severe sway while testing the Romberg's sign. The finger to nose test, rapid hand acceleration, heel down the shin, and past pointing were all decreased on her left. All of her orthopedic tests were positive, including her range of motion in her neck and lower back.

After treating her for seven months, **all** of her conditions improved. She no longer suffered from headaches, tremors, back pain, or leg pain. Paula Jean wrote this letter to her insurance company when a medical doctor stated that she had "reached maximum medical improvement" and the insurance company refused to pay any longer once her lower back pain had subsided:

While it is true that I began seeing Dr. Johnson with the only complaint being back pain, as I began treatment, I noticed that Dr. Johnson was helping some other problems I had just learned to live with and hadn't even told the doctor about at the initial evaluation. Sometimes you don't notice things have improved until they are gone because you have accepted them as normal. Headaches, poor balance, and tremors in the hands are all symptoms that I have lived with for a long time. All of the symptoms improved with the treatment provided by Dr. Johnson. As I let Dr. Johnson know these things, treatments were changed and added. I had some dizziness that returned, but it has cleared up. My balance is improving, as well as the hand tremors. It would be worth it to get off the medication that I take monthly for the tremors. The headaches now occur every other month instead of weekly or daily. Dr. Johnson has not given up and feels that we can resolve it further.

Sincerely,
   Paula Jean

Lana
History:

This 50 year-old female presented to my office in May of 1999 complaining of pain and stiffness throughout her entire body. She stated that she suffered from a dull ache from her head down to her toes. She was very fatigued and suffered from irritable bowel syndrome. She stated that a simple touch, a piece of clothing, or a pat on the back would be unbelievably painful to her. She wore slacks that were two sizes too big so that they wouldn't touch her body. Lana would spend one to three hours a day taking hot baths to obtain some relief. Any change in routine where she was unable to eat or sleep on a regular schedule, such as taking a trip, would trigger problems to the point where her symptoms would be multiplied for weeks on end. Riding in the car was virtually impossible. Lana also told me that one day, while raking her lawn, her heart rate increased from a normal rate of 75 beats per minute to 200 beats per minute and continued at that level for over three hours. She reported that she had suffered from tachycardia (increased heart rate) for many years.

Lana also found it very difficult to concentrate. Any distraction would make her lose her place or forget what she was doing. (A lack of concentration is due to a lack of impulses, or frequency of firing, in the temporal lobe, specifically the right temporal lobe.) It was difficult for Lana to carry on a conversation if there was any background noise, such as a radio or TV. She had also become extremely sensitive to smell, light, and sound. Sleep was almost nonexistent for Lana, which resulted in an extremely low energy level. Many nights the pain would wake her up after only two or three hours of sleep, even though she had taken strong medications to help her sleep. She would arise at approximately 2:00 A.M. and take a hot bath to relieve some of the pain. At one point, her doctor ordered total bed rest for a week due to her severe low back pain.

Even though Lana suffered as she did, she seldom missed work because she had to support her family. Many times, her husband would have to help her from the street to the sidewalk after work, as she couldn't make the step alone. Simple things, such as opening an office or bathroom door, were difficult. After work each day, she would spend approximately 90 minutes in a bath so she could relax her muscles and attempt to get some sleep. She would then eat, take her medication, and retire for the night.

Lana had been treated by doctor after doctor for over twenty-five years. She had been on a number of medications; her prescription would change with every "miracle" medication that came onto the market. In the past, medical doctors told her to exercise and completely eliminate all caffeine. She explained to the doctors that exercise was difficult because of the extreme pain throughout her body. The doctors told her to "get off her butt" and do it anyway. I frequently hear this statement from chronic pain patients. Their spouses, medical doctors, or healing practitioners will tell them to simply eat right and exercise. If they did, they wouldn't be in such a predicament. "Your pain can't be that bad," many are told.

Every test that I performed on Lana was positive. I explained to Lana that this would be a long, hard road back, but we could definitely help her with her condition. By the sixth week of treatments, Lana's pain and fatigue were much improved. I then had to go out of town for a neurology conference and had an associate cover for me. Unfortunately, the associate didn't pay attention to Lana's file. I specifically stated that no structural adjustments (popping or cracking) were to be performed on Lana due to her compromised nervous system. He administered a structural adjustment to Lana's cervical spine anyway. What many doctors do not realize is that you can make people well with manipulation, but you can also make them worse. You have to adjust the treatment modality in accordance to the specific patient because each patient has his/her own specific baseline of his/her nervous system. This baseline is called the central integrated state or CIS. Not every patient will tolerate structural adjustment, just as not every patient would feel the benefit of a low force adjustment such as an activator. This was a major setback for Lana, but she stuck through the treatments. Over time, she continued to see improvements to the point where she has written the following testimonial:

11/20/99

As Thanksgiving Day approaches, I think of how thankful I am that my health has improved since Apple Medical Clinic started treating me. Before coming to Apple Medical Clinic, I had to eat the same limited diet, exercise the same, and go to bed at the same time or my problems would get worse. I also could do very little physically. I hadn't vacuumed or even picked up sticks in the yard for years.

Since coming to Apple Medical Clinic for treatment, my health no longer controls my life. I can vacuum, rake leaves, even take two-day bus trips and have few negative health problems. I appreciate being able to do things again. A simple thing like waking up in the morning and being able to stretch or stand without pain is something I never dreamed would happen again. Thanks for improving the quality of my life!

I'm also thankful for Apple Medical Clinic treating their patients as individuals. It is so helpful to be able to feel comfortable to tell them small things that cause me discomfort, knowing they won't make light of them.

Thank you,
Lana

Lana <u>BEFORE TX</u>

First thing I feel in the morning is pain.

I couldn't stand up straight for a length of time in the morning-sometimes hours.

Since 1974, from my waist down I often felt achy, numb, and tingly, especially one week of the month. I took 8 special supplements a day that helped some-if I tried taking less the aching got worse. My legs often ached so badly that I would often rub or massage them as fast as I sat.
Spent about 1 1/2 hours every night taking a hot bath before I went to bed so my muscles wouldn't hurt and I could sleep.

Sometimes I would still wake up with pain after 4 or 5 hours of sleep and take another hot bath before I went to work.

Had problems with tachycardia most of my life. Until the last 8 years I would lie down and it would go away and there would be no side effects. The last 8 years I often had a problem getting my heart to slow back down. 3 or 4 times after having a pulse of 200 for about 2 hours I would go to the emergency room. After these long episodes it would often take me 1 to 4 weeks to have my energy level back to normal.

Lana after TX:

The first thing I do in the morning is stretch and NO PAIN.

I can stand up straight right away in the morning or within a few steps.

I seldom have any achy numb feeling from the waist down. One week of the month I may have it slightly. Since July 1999, I've been off all 8 supplements I took for this problem.

I can sleep without taking a hot bath.

I only woke up with pain once in the past several months.

I've only had three episodes with tachycardia since May 1999. Twice it only lasted a few minutes and once it went away as soon as I lay down. I had no side effects after these episodes.

Janie
History:

Janie, a 35 year-old-female, had been suffering with chronic fatigue and fibromyalgia for four years. She had been diagnosed by a rheumatologist and had been under the care of many medical doctors before presenting to my office. Upon presentation, Janie was taking the medication Amitriptyline to help her sleep and Ibuprofen for the pain. She had been suffering from severe headaches and dizziness for the past five years. She stated that she had a low-grade headache everyday and a migraine headache occasionally.

She noticed visual changes during her migraine headaches, and she fatigued very easily. Her head felt so heavy that she was having difficulty holding it up, and when she turned her head, she would become dizzy and nauseous.

Janie also suffered from severe cognitive problems. Many people call it a "brain fog," and I find that many fibromyalgia patients suffer from it. She stated that it felt like she was in a fog; she had difficulty recalling information and finding the right word to say. She wasn't able to follow instructions due to a complete lack of focus. When speaking, she would trail off in mid-sentence. She also suffered from memory loss. When she was driving to certain places, she would forget where she was going and would take the wrong turn. She felt as if she was dyslexic because she would write things down incorrectly. At the time, she was in school, and she would transfer test answers incorrectly to the score sheet. She would throw things away that she should have kept, prepare food incorrectly, put items away and forget where they were, and repeat herself over and over. She was unable to remember phone numbers and specific dates, and she had difficulty adding and subtracting. When reading, she would have to read paragraphs three to four times, and even then she had a difficult time remembering what she had read. Many times she would simply sit in a daze thinking about nothing.

Janie's eyes and mouth were dry constantly. Her neck was very painful, and the pain radiated up into her right ear. She found it hard to swallow at times and choked very easily. Her arms and legs were extremely weak, and she felt pain in all her joints and muscles. Her pain sensation was heightened to the point that jeans irritated her skin. Janie would suffer daily from cramps and twitching throughout her entire body. She also noticed that when sitting for an extended period, she would experience numbness on her entire right side.

Janie experienced abdominal pain daily and had difficulty with her bowel movements. At times, she would experience constipation, at other times, diarrhea. She also experienced episodes of frequent urination. Her heart rate was very high and she had difficulty taking deep breaths. Balance problems also plagued her - she would often walk into walls and doorways. She was very sensitive to light, and she noticed that in the previous six months, she had experienced an increase in sweating. She had trouble getting to sleep, and when she woke up at night, she was unable to get back to sleep. She noticed that lately she had been more irritable and had experienced episodes of depression and anxiety.

In 1997, she had been released from work to a disability status. She was also a student carrying twelve credits, but she reduced her load to six credits because of her condition.

Examination:

Upon examination, I found several problems consistent with other fibromyalgia patients, including a large left pupil, a decrease in the optokinetic tape testing on the left, a left palatal paresis, and a left ptosis. I observed a severe sway when Janie stood with her feet together and eyes closed. She exhibited decreased finger to nose and rapid hand acceleration on the right. When moving her right heel down her left shin, I observed shaking, which indicated a decrease in impulses of the lateral, or outer aspect, of the cerebellum.

I began a treatment protocol of very light adjustments on the right upper and lower extremities and an activator adjustment on the cervical spine. Oxygen was administered per our medical director since oxygen cannot be administered by a chiropractor in the State of Wisconsin. Eventually, I administered T.E.N.S. (electrical stimulation) and heat on her right arm and right shoulder to increase the frequency of firing, or impulses, to the right cerebellum and left-brain. Within the first two weeks, Janie started to notice that her symptoms were slightly improving. After approximately six to eight weeks, her symptoms had greatly improved. She continued with care until she experienced some financial setbacks and was forced to discontinue care. She stated that when she was able to, she would return to care.

I saw Janie in the bakery a while back, and she stated that she was still doing quite well. I don't know what she was doing in the bakery - she shouldn't have been there, but then again, I shouldn't have been there either. It's hard to judge what someone else should eat when you are walking out of the bakery with two dozen cinnamon rolls.

Laura
History:

Laura, a 34 year-old female, presented to Apple Medical Clinic with extreme fatigue, neck, shoulder, and arm pain, headaches, lower back pain, and leg pain. She stated that she had been suffering from this condition for approximately five years. She had been experiencing migraine headaches to the point where she would become very nauseated, and she suffered from extreme light sensitivity. She had difficulty sleeping and noticed that she was becoming more irritable and angry. Laura had been on numerous medications over the past five years; her Amitriptyline did allow her to sleep five hours per night. She was also given Imitrex as needed for the migraine headaches, which provided her with some relief. She had been under the care of two chiropractors and three medical doctors before presenting to our office.

Examination:

Tissue saturation of oxygen was within normal limits. Her initial examination was unremarkable except for a decrease in left optokinetic tape testing and a severe left exophoria. Orthopedic tests were all positive. In healthcare, positive means bad and negative means good. Go figure?

Treatment for Laura's condition was visual and auditory stimulation and adjustments on the right side only. Auditory stimulation consisted of ocean sounds in the right ear for approximately ten minutes, and visual stimulation consisted of red and black squares at approximately 2 hertz on the left side.

After about twelve visits, Laura had made remarkable improvement. After six weeks and eighteen visits, she was re-examined, and she found that her pain symptoms had decreased by fifty percent. She presented with a pain intensity of "9" on the 0-10 pain scale, but after six weeks of treatment, her pain was at a "4" along with good objective changes.

We continued to treat Laura in a similar manner; along with adjustments on the right side, visual stimulation, and auditory stimulation, we added T.E.N.S. (electrical stimulation), vibration, and an occasional caloric. After three months of treatment, Laura was symptom-free. I continue to see her on a bi-monthly basis and have given her eye exercises to increase the function of her cerebellum. Laura now uses a squeeze ball in the right hand to increase the function of the nucleus, or outside, of the cerebellum. She also uses different types of brainteasers, including word searches and mazes, to increase the frequency of firing of specific parts of the brain.

Guaifenesin

Guaifenesin is a medication that was developed to treat high uric acid levels (gout) and nasal congestion.

In the past few years, some medical doctors have been prescribing Guaifenesin for patients suffering from fibromyalgia. Their theory is that fibromyalgia patients are unable to eliminate excess uric acid from their bodies.

I have treated fibromyalgia patients in which Guaifenesin has helped tremendously and others where it provided absolutely no relief. The symptoms of fibromyalgia may become worse when initiating Guaifenesin, but will eventually subside.

Should fibromyalgia patients give Guaifenesin a try?

Certainly! I'm for anything that will help relieve chronic, debilitating health conditions.

(Please note that the preceding case histories are only a few of the thousands of patients that we have helped in our clinic in the past 20 years.)

Chapter 9:
Other Chronic Conditions

"The head of medical service in a great university hospital once said, 'One should send for his minister (or priest or rabbi) as he sends for his doctor when he becomes ill.' That is to say, God helps the sick in two ways, through the science of medicine and surgery and through the science of faith and prayer."
-Norman Vincent Peale: *Today*

My purpose in listing all of these case histories is to point out the fact that every patient must be treated as an individual. There should be no "cookie cutter" treatment modality used in the same way for every patient. In our office, three patients may be treated with auditory stimulation, but all three may receive different frequencies. In many cases, doctors will become accustomed using a specific treatment modality, and they will use only that modality on every patient who walks into the office.

I am amazed to see how many doctors - whether they are chiropractors, medical doctors, or osteopaths - give up on the patient who suffers from a chronic condition. Perhaps if the doctor had suffered as the patient does, he would not give up so easily.

Marlene

History:

Marlene, a 63 year-old female, presented to my office in severe pain. She had been suffering from sciatica (leg pain) of the left leg for the previous few weeks. The pain was so severe that she was forced to use a walker. Marlene had been under the treatment of another chiropractor with limited results. Six months before presenting to my office, she had surgery on her lower back in an attempt to relieve her sciatica. Following the surgery, the pain had switched from her left leg to her right leg. Her orthopedic surgeon recommended exercise and stated that the pain would go away in a month or two. It didn't. After about six weeks of suffering with severe left sciatica, Marlene hobbled into my office. It was virtually impossible to examine Marlene due to the severity of the pain that she was experiencing, but her vitals did show an extreme decrease in her tissue saturation of oxygen. Marlene was administer oxygen per direct order from our medical doctor. Oxygen is fuel to the brain just as gas is to the car. If the car does not have any gas, you cannot drive anywhere. If the brain does not have fuel, you can do all of the treatments you want, but you will not help the patient.

Examination:

Marlene exhibited a left exophoria upon accommodation, a decreased optokinetic tape test on the left, and a left palatal paresis.

She was unable to perform Romberg's sign. She also exhibited decreased muscle strength in the left upper extremity. Based on these findings, I decided to adjust Marlene on her right side on a daily basis. The first few visits were extremely difficult for Marlene, but by her fourth visit, her pain intensity was a "5."

This was a significant improvement considering that upon initial presentation her pain level was a "10" with "0" being no pain and "10 being very severe pain. We continued to treat Marlene, and by the end of her eighteen-visit treatment trial, Marlene was free of pain.

Lawrence

History:

This 68 year-old male presented to my office complaining of pain in the left hip and left leg for well over 20 years that started when he was a school bus driver. He stated that the pain was constant but varied in intensity, and it seemed to be worse when he woke up in the morning. He had been under the care of medical doctors and chiropractors over the years; some gave him relief, but some were "a big waste of my time," as Lawrence put it.

Examination:

Upon examination of Lawrence, I found a decreased tissue saturation of oxygen, a decrease in muscle strength in the left upper extremity, a decrease in right olfactory perception, a decrease in right optokinetic tape testing, a severe right exophoria, a facial paresis on the left, and a right palatal paresis. During the Romberg's sign and Tandem walk tests, Lawrence exhibited a severe sway.

I chose to adjust the left side of Lawrence's body to increase the frequency of firing to the left cerebellum. T.E.N.S. (Transcutaneous electronic nerve stimulation) and vibration were administered on this left side. Vibration increases the frequency of firing, or impulses, to the cerebellum via the dorsal columns (back part of the spinal cord). In addition to these treatment modalities, we administered oxygen, per direct order from our medical director because Lawrence's tissue saturation of oxygen was so depleted.

After suffering with debilitating hip and leg pain for over 20 years and having been treated by a multitude of doctors, I am happy to report that after his first treatment trial of eighteen visits, Lawrence was completely pain-free. Because his was such a chronic condition, I treated Lawrence a little further, then dismissed him to a PRN status. I happened to see Lawrence downtown last week, and when I asked him how he was, he said that he had "never felt better." Lawrence told me that he was very thankful for the help our office provided him.

"My Hip and leg Pain Are Gone"

For the last 15 years, I have suffered from pain in my hips and aches in my legs. The pain would start at the top of my left leg and radiate down the entire leg into my foot. The pain continued to worsen so I had an MRI which revealed a deteriorated disc which was pinching off the nerve in my left leg. I underwent surgery to remove the disc. It didn't help. I thought that I would have to live with the pain the rest of my life.

I saw an ad for Apple Medical Clinic and called for an appointment. I felt that I had nothing to lose.

I have been receiving treatment at Apple Medical Clinic which has resulted in a huge improvement in my hips and legs. My hip and leg pain is gone!

Lawrence

Corrine

History:

This 72 year-old female presented to my office complaining of numbness in both feet. She stated that the numbness had been bothering her for the past seven years. Medical doctors, neurologists, podiatrists, chiropractors, and physical therapists had all treated Corrine unsuccessfully. She was prescribed many medications, including Neurontin, that provided no relief. The physical therapist had given Corrine exercises that provided some degree of relief in the beginning, but the relief did not continue. She stated that the numbness was primarily under the ball of the foot on both sides, and she described the feeling as a "rolled up sock was under her toes."

Examination:

Examination revealed a decrease in pinwheel sensation and vibration sensation on the left side in the upper and lower extremities. A decrease in the muscle stretch reflexes, a left exophoria upon accommodation, a left corectasia, a decrease in the left opto-kinetic tape testing, and a left palatal paresis were also noted. When standing with her feet together and eyes closed (Romberg's sign), Corrine would sway violently from side to side. When touching her finger to her nose, she missed with her right hand. Rapid hand acceleration and past pointing were decreased on the right. A severe muscle spasm was noted in the lumbar spine, and a mild to moderate muscle spasm was observed throughout the cervical and thoracic spine. Corrine's tissue saturation of oxygen was very low, at 92-93%; normal tissue saturation of oxygen is usually 98-100%. Many medical doctors insist that anything above 90% is normal, and that is fine from a cardiovascular standpoint. From a neurological standpoint, oxygen is fuel to the brain and nervous system, and we would like the oxygen level as high as possible.

Treatment for Corrine consisted of manipulations to the right side of the body, moist heat to the cervical spine to increase the frequency of firing to the right cerebellum, electrical stimulation on the right side, and treatment of multiple food allergies. After Corrine's initial treatment of six weeks, the intensity of her numbness went from a "10" to a "7," with "0" corresponding to no numbness and "10" corresponding to severe numbness. At that point, we performed multiple subjective tests during a re-examination. After a twelve-week treatment trial, Corrine's numbness intensity was down to a "4." This was the first improvement in her numbness with any type of doctor in the past seven years. I continue to treat Corrine on a weekly basis, and presently her numbness intensity is down to a "2."

Maxine

History:

Maxine, a 66 year-old female, presented to my office complaining of pain in her right hip, lower back, and left leg. Maxine came to my office after hearing a speech I performed at a Multiple Sclerosis support group meeting. She has had MS for years and has been under the care of a medical neurologist for as long as she has suffered with MS. Maxine stated that she also suffered from headaches that would start at the back of her neck and radiate up into the frontal aspect of her head. At the time of presentation, Maxine was on the medications Avenex, Avioennex, Accuretic, and Actonel.

Examination:

Upon examination of Maxine, I found a decrease in the muscle stretch reflexes, a definite decrease in the muscle strength of the lower left extremity, and a left ptosis (the eyelid is much lower than the opposite eyelid). A left corectasia was noted, and Maxine exhibited a marked decrease in the optokinetic tape test when moving the tape to the left. I observed a left exophoria, a left palatal paresis, and a left hypoglossal nerve - in this case, her tongue deviated to the left. Maxine fell straight backward while testing the Romberg's sign and exhibited a decrease in the right rapid hand acceleration.

I chose to adjust the right side of Maxine's body to increase frequency of firing to the same-side cerebellum via stimulation of muscle, joint, and tendon receptors, which in turn would stimulate large diameter nerves. Maxine received electrical stimulation on the right side, and she received vibration stimulation to increase the frequency of firing to the back part of the spinal cord (dorsal columns). After a six-week treatment trial, Maxine stated that her pain was 40-50% improved. More importantly, many of her objective findings improved. Therefore, I knew that I was making permanent changes in her nervous system. After sixteen weeks of care, Maxine was completely free of pain for the first time in a long time. Maxine stated that this was the first time in recent memory she had been absolutely symptom-free.

Ed:

History:

Ed, a 68-year-old male, presented to my clinic complaining of low back pain, leg pain, and numbness in his arms and legs. Ed stated that he had been suffering from this condition for the past thirty years. Ed's level of pain would often vary between an 8 and 10, with 0 being no pain at all and 10 being very severe pain. He stated that his numbness would be worse in the morning and seemed to "ease up" as the day went on. Throughout his thirty years of suffering, Ed had endured three back surgeries and one surgery on his cervical spine (neck). Five years ago Ed had become addicted to pain medication and had been through detoxification twice. At the time of presentation he stated that he was not taking any type of prescription medication, but was taking over the counter medication such as Tylenol and Advil. Ed had been referred by another patient of mine. He was not very optimistic, but was willing to give it a shot since his friend had such good results.

Examination:

The examination revealed a decrease in the tissue saturation of oxygen. Ed's tissue saturation of oxygen on the left side was 90%, and on the right side was 92%. Normal tissue saturation of oxygen is 98 to 100%. His chest expansion was only 1/2 inch, his salivary pH level was 5.5. His muscle stretch reflexes were all diminished and he had a slight weakness in muscle strength on his left side. Vibratory and pinwheel sensation were equal bilaterally. He had a slight arrythmia when auscultating his heart. A severe blepherospasm was noted with a decrease in left olfactory perception. When moving the optokinetic tape to the left there was a decrease in the slow parietal pursuit. There was a severe left exophoria upon accommodation. When standing with his feet together and eyes closed Ed exhibited a severe global sway. All of the orthopedic tests on Ed's lower back were positive. X-rays revealed rather severe osteoarthritis or degenerative changes in the lower lumbar spine.

I told Ed that I wasn't going to make him any promises, but I would do my very best to help him and that my normal treatment protocol with all patients is a six week treatment trial of three times per week. After conferring with our medical director, she and I reviewed Ed's file and agreed that Ed's tissue saturation of oxygen was very low and that administering oxygen would benefit him greatly. If you remember in my previous chapters I had stated that the brain needs two things to survive, fuel and activation, fuel being oxygen and glucose.

By the third week Ed stated that he was feeling somewhat better and by the sixth week Ed's pain was down to a five, with zero being no pain and ten being severe pain. At the end of a twelve week treatment protocol, Ed's pain was now down to a 3. He stated that it was the best he had felt in thirty years. At the end of sixteen weeks, Ed's pain was down to a 2, and the numbness was almost gone. In addition to improved subjective findings (symptoms), a re-examination of Ed revealed remarkable improvement in objective findings (tests). Ed stated that the numbness would return if he chopped wood or overextend himself by lifting heavy objects. Overall Ed was ecstatic about his recovery.

Kathleen:

History:

Kathleen, a 45-year-old housewife, presented to my office complaining of headaches, light headedness, and neck pain which radiated down into her shoulders. Kathleen had suffered from this condition approximately four years. Kathleen stated that her pain level was a 7, with 0 being no pain and 10 being very severe pain. Three years prior Kathleen had undergone neck surgery, in which plates and screws had been inserted into her cervical spine from the level of C4 to C7 (see figure 9-1). She stated that the surgery had provided her with some degree of relief, but not the permanent relief she was seeking.

Examination:

Upon examination of Kathleen I found a mild blepherospasm, a right corectasia, a decrease in the right slow parietal pursuits, fast frontal refixation saccade, and contralateral cerebellar termination utilizing the optokinetic tape. She had a severe right exophoria, a right palatal paresis, a moderate sway when standing with her feet together and eyes closed, and positive orthopedic and neurological tests.

I began to treat Kathleen utilizing oxygen, manual adjustments, and T.E.N.S., and I am very happy to report that four months after her initial treatment had begun, Kathleen's pain level is now a 1, with 0 being no pain and 10 being very severe pain.

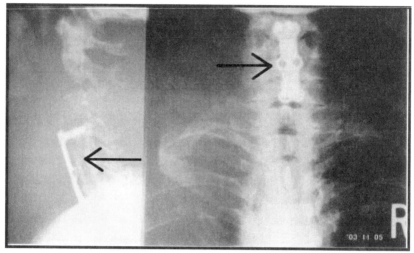

Figure 9-1

(Please note that the preceding case histories are only a few of the thousands of patients that we have helped in our clinic in the past 20 years.)

Chapter 10:
Chiropractic and Strokes

"The health of the people is really the foundation upon which all their happiness and all their powers as a state depend."
-Benjamin Disrael

On May 20, 2003, a press release was issued regarding manipulations of the cervical spine, or neck, and strokes. The press release involved an article in the medical journal *Neurology*. The article stated that cervical manipulations may cause strokes and that those practitioners providing these types of manipulations should be very cautious.

In the Canadian paper *The Post* dated July of 2000, an article titled "Chiropractic Neck Manipulations Linked to Strokes" by Mary Vallus also pointed out that cervical manipulations may cause strokes. Naturally, chiropractors disagreed with these findings for a variety of reasons.

Personally, I am aware of at least five strokes that have been caused by chiropractic manipulations since 1990 in the state of Wisconsin. I have had a number of patients present to my office complaining of headaches, blurred vision, nausea, and dizziness after receiving bilateral cervical spine (neck) manipulations from chiropractors.

Unfortunately, many patients that I have treated, who have been under the care of previous chiropractors, have not had a thorough physical examination or x-rays with the advent of the HMOs. A thorough examination is <u>extremely</u> important to determine if the patient's cervical spine (neck) should be manipulated or adjusted. If a patient presents with numerous signs of cranial nerve malfunctions such as a large pupil (3rd cranial nerve), exophoria upon accommodation (4th cranial nerve), positive corneal reflex (5th and 7th cranial nerve), facial paresis (7th cranial nerve) along with a high output of the mesencephalic pools (increased sweating, light sensitivity, increased heart rate, inability to sleep, difficulty urinating, and/or constipation), the doctor should not perform a cervical spine (neck) manipulation or adjustment. Chiropractors who sign on with HMOs are paid on a capitation basis, meaning that the chiropractor has an "x" amount of patients and is paid a "y" amount for those patients whether they see him/her or not. Sadly, these chiropractors have cut corners to save costs, and they have elected not to provide a thorough examination and x-rays. As a result, many patients are suffering severe consequences.

The following is a portion of an article that appeared in the *Journal of the American Chiropractic Association* titled "Iatrogenesis in Medical and Chiropractic Interventions: A Thumbnail Cost Analysis."

1. Chiropractic death rate = 3 per 10 million manipulations.
2. ASSUME: average number of manipulations/patient = 10.
3. Total number of chiropractic office visits nationwide = 250million/year.
   a. So annual number of patient-episodes treated each year by chiropractors= 250 million divided by 10 = 25 million.
4. Number of patients treated for neck and cervical problems each year = 42% x 25 million = 10.5 million.
5. So annual number of patients lost to arterial dissection (tearing of the artery in the neck) = 10.5 million x 3 divided by 10 million = 3.
6. Annual death rate due to medication = 79,000 – 400,000, costing $76.6 billion nationwide.
   a. So arterial dissection death rate = 10.5 million x 3 divided by 10 million (0.0038-0.00075% the corresponding rates obtained with medications).
7. If we reduce the use of medication by just 15%, by extrapolation, cut drug-related morbidity/mortality costs by $11.5 billion.
8. Using chiropractic office charge of $45, nationwide cost of annual number of adjustments (250 million) calculates to $11.25 billion.
9. Therefore, reduction of medication use by 15% would more than pay for the total bill of chiropractic services to all Americans at the current rate of utilization.
   a. Theoretically, would save anywhere from 11,850-60,000 lives.
   b. Would also save all legal costs and man-hours lost to litigation relating to drug-related morbidity.

The article states that the chiropractic death rate is 3 per 10 million manipulations and the number of manipulations is 250 million per year. Using these figures, 75 deaths result from chiropractic manipulations each year. The article goes on to state that the annual death rate due to medication is 79,000-400,000 per year. This is an unfortunate comparison in that chiropractors are always pointing fingers at medical doctors and medical doctors will continue to point fingers at chiropractors. In my opinion, chiropractors need to police chiropractors and medical doctors need to police medical doctors. The patient is in the middle and is the one losing out.

The fact is that 75 people die because of chiropractic manipulations each year. An estimated 250 have strokes, but the exact number is not known because the chiropractic malpractice insurance companies (including mine – NCMIC-National Chiropractic Mutual Insurance Company) refuse to release this data. The probability of a stroke is 1 per 1 million manipulations, and when 250 million manipulations are performed each year, it does not take a rocket scientist to figure out that about 250 people suffer strokes each year as a direct result of cervical (neck) manipulations. Although the odds seem very low (one in a million), what happens if **you** win the lottery?

The last stroke directly caused by a chiropractor that I am aware of was approximately 3 miles from my office, in the summer of 2001. A 42 year-old male suffered a severe stroke on the chiropractor's table after receiving a cervical (neck) manipulation. The case was taken to court, and the plaintiff (patient) was awarded $250,000 by the jury. To this day, the chiropractor continues to practice.

Because of this stroke incident, I began a letter-writing campaign explaining how important it is for chiropractors to perform a thorough examination, otherwise, very serious consequences could result. I have sent letters to various health plans, regulating agencies, and associations. Not one of these agencies responded to my call for increased awareness of strokes caused by manipulation. I even sent a letter to Russ Leonard, the executive director of the Wisconsin Chiropractic Association. Mr. Leonard never responded, probably because he was busy with other endeavors.

In 2001, Russ Leonard was convicted of price fixing by the

Wisconsin Department of Justice. Even with the conviction, the WCA Board of Directors continue to wholeheartedly support him. I guess, in the state of Wisconsin, illegal activity done on the behalf of the Wisconsin Chiropractic Association further endears you to the chiropractic community.

My advice to potential patients is "consumer beware." If a patient presents to a doctor with positive neurological findings like those I have mentioned in previous chapters, it is probably within the best interest of the patient not to manipulate the cervical spine or the neck region. If the doctor fails to perform a thorough and comprehensive examination prior to treatment get up and run out of the office.

Chapter 11:
Nutrition

"A wise man should consider that health is the greatest of human blessings, and learn how by his own thought to derne benefit from his illness."

-Hippocrates

Over the past twenty years, I have attended numerous nutrition seminars and have read countless nutrition books. All of this does not necessarily make me an expert, but at least I have some nutritional background. Most medical doctors and some chiropractors do not study nutrition, but they simply refer their patients to a registered dietitian. A registered dietitian may or may not agree with what I am about to tell you, but after treating patients for over twenty years, this program has worked for hundreds of my patients.

I personally take a daily multivitamin and essential fatty acids, or EFAs (Omega-3, Omega-6). I also take 1000-1500 mg of calcium, depending on my diet that week. If I eat more dairy products, I will take less calcium, and vice versa. I try to eat as much organically grown food as possible. Meat, dairy, and eggs all contain small amounts of hormones and antibiotics that were given to the animals. Fruits and vegetables contain pesticide residues. Organically produced food may cost more, but you get what you pay for. I have a very low caffeine intake, meaning that if I do drink coffee or soda, I will only drink decaffeinated. My sugar intake is low to moderate, my protein intake is high, my alcohol intake is very low, and my carbohydrate intake is low to moderate. I try to drink 1/2 of my body weight in ounces of water per day. This way, even if I don't reach my goal, I at least get the minimum recommendation (64 oz.) of water per day. It's extremely important to keep yourself hydrated. The book entitled, *Your Body's Many Cries for Water* by Fereydoon Batmanghelidj, M.D., and *The Shocking Truth About Water* by Paul Bragg, are both great reads.

I exercise daily for 45 minutes to 1 hour and vary my program between weights, walking/running, and the UBE. I realize that patients suffering from severe dizziness, fibromyalgia, or migraine headaches cannot exercise due to their symptoms. Once I've helped these patients with their condition, I start them on a light exercise program of walking and then work up from that point.

Exercise invigorates the brain! It increases the brain's frequency of firing or impulses. Remember, a healthy brain equals a healthy life.

Calcium

Calcium is not only essential for the development and maintenance of healthy bones and teeth, but it also helps maintain cell membranes, connective tissue, and normal blood pressure. You hear everyone talking today about which source of calcium is the best, whether it is coral calcium, powdered calcium, or calcium in tablet form. Calcium comes in many forms, including carbonate, citrate, aspartame, glutamate, escorbate, and bone meal. When it comes to nutrition, my advice is to keep it simple. The only type of calcium that I recommend is calcium citrate. Calcium citrate is 24% calcium, and it is well absorbed. Plus, it reduces the risk of kidney stones and is absorbed by those with poor digestion. Calcium carbonate, which is the cheapest and most popular source of calcium, is not a complete bone food. It may be malabsorbed by those with poor stomach digestion, and it has an antacid affect, which is why you will see calcium carbonate in products like *TUMS*. The antacid affect may actually interfere with digestion and cause gas. Bone meal is 39% calcium, but it may contain high amounts of lead, arsenic, or cadmium. The heating process used to form the calcium tablet also substantially destroys its organic constituency. I simply recommend to my patients that they take calcium citrate at approximately 1,000 to 1,500 mg per day, depending on the individual patient. Whole foods are the best sources of calcium - and all other nutrients - as the body can better absorb calcium from food. The calcium is also accompanied by other essential nutrients, including fiber, antioxidants, and protein.

Good food sources of calcium: Broccoli, cheeses, collard greens, corn tortillas (processed with lime), kale, milk (fat-free), mustard greens, orange juice (fortified), salmon with bones (canned), sardines with bones, and yogurt (fat-free).

Essential Fatty Acids
(Omega-6 and Omega-3 oils)

Omega-3 essential fatty acids are found in fatty deep water fish, like salmon and tuna, and Omega-6 essential fatty acids are found in vegetable oils, including safflower, black currant, and evening primrose. A deficiency in essential fatty acids will cause dry or rough skin and brittle nails, and in women, it will cause menstrual cramps. EFAs are also vital for the function of your body's outer membrane, your skin.

Omega-3 essential fatty acids are necessary for normal activity of nerve tissue. Along with B vitamins and amino acids, essential fatty acids are very important for the proper function of the brain, brainstem, spinal cord (central nervous system), and peripheral nervous system (outlying nerves). The cell wall of the neuron, or nerve cell, is made up of lipoproteins, fats (lipo-) and proteins. In the past few years, many patients have become concerned about their cholesterol levels. Cholesterol isn't the only thing patients should be concerned with. Patients should be equally concerned with high-density lipids (HDL's), low-density lipids (LDL's), and tryglicerides. High cholesterol levels, high trygliceride levels, and high levels of low-density lipids have all been linked to a diet high in non-essential fats, or saturated fats. Studies have shown that when patients increase their intake of essential fatty acids, their trygliceride levels, cholesterol levels, and blood pressure fall. Essential fatty acids trigger the production of prostaglandins that dilate, or enlarge, the blood vessels and make the blood less sticky. A diet high in saturated fat - one including lots of fried foods and red meat - leads to the development of hypertension and arteriosclerosis. By replacing saturated fats with essential fatty acids, patients will experience positive effects in their cardiovascular system.

A recent study by the National Institute of Mental Health (NIMH), revealed "The brain is composed of lipids and fatty acids, so it makes perfect sense that EFA's will increase a patient's mental well being."

Good food sources of EFAs: Cold water fish (especially tuna and salmon), nuts (especially almonds and walnuts), and flaxseed, safflower, black currant, and evening primrose oils.

Magnesium

Magnesium is necessary for healthy heart function and the conversion of carbohydrates, fats, and proteins into energy. It also helps in the manufacturing of proteins and synthesis of genetic material within each cell. Magnesium supports muscle relaxation, muscle contraction, and nerve transmission. When my patients suffer from twitching muscles, I often find that they suffer from magnesium deficiency.

Good food sources of magnesium: Avocados, bananas, broccoli, brown rice, haddock, navy beans, oatmeal, pinto beans, spinach, sweet potatoes, and yogurt.

Selenium

Selenium plays an important role as a component of the antioxidant enzyme glutathioneperoxidase. Some studies have shown that patients suffering from rheumatoid arthritis have lower levels of selenium in their blood. Selenium also has many antioxidant properties.

Good food sources of selenium: Clams, crab, lobster, oysters (cooked), and whole grains.

Zinc

Zinc is a component of numerous enzymes and plays a role in protein synthesis. It also helps to balance blood sugar and heal wounds, and it is necessary for proper brain function. Zinc maintains healthy skin, the immune system, and the nervous, digestive, and reproductive systems, and it is an important antioxidant in that it protects white blood cells. A zinc deficiency impairs the immune function and predisposes a patient to infection. It is important to note that diets too high in iron and calcium block the body's absorption of zinc, and one sign of a zinc deficiency is white spots on a patient's fingernails.

Good food sources of zinc: Beef, eggs, lamb, nuts, oysters (cooked), whole grains, and yogurt.

Vitamin A

Vitamin A maintains normal eyesight, helps the immune system response, allows for embryonic development, and maintains tissues that line the bodies internal and external surfaces.

Good food sources for vitamin A: Butternut squash, cantaloupe, carrot juice, carrots, mangoes, pumpkins, spinach, sweet potatoes, and tuna.

Vitamin B1

B1 plays a major role in the conversion of protein, fats, and carbohydrates to energy. B1 also aids detoxification and heart and nervous system function. B vitamins should never be taken individually, and if you need to take B1, make sure to take it with a multivitamin or B complex. Taking a B vitamin individually may cause a deficiency with other B vitamins.

Good food sources of vitamin B1: Avocado, beans, broccoli, cherries, garlic, and alfalfa sprouts.

Vitamin B2

B2 is essential for cellular energy production. It supports hormone production, healthy eyes and skin, and the production of red blood cells. It also supports the function of neurotransmitters, chemicals that allow your nerves to communicate with one another.

Good food sources of vitamin B2: Bananas, cashews, apples, almonds, asparagus, and apricots.

Vitamin B6

B6 is essential for protein synthesis and the manufacture of hormones, red blood cells and enzymes. Vitamin B6 plays an important role in hormone regulation, brain function, skin health, and is crucial for a healthy immune system. It should be noted that the nervous system and the immune system function together as one. Many doctors don't realize that when they observe a compromised immune system, they are actually observing a compromised nervous system.

Good food sources vitamin B6: Avocados, bananas, beef, brewer's yeast, brown rice, chicken, eggs, oats, peanuts, soybeans, walnuts, and whole wheat.

Vitamin B12

Vitamin B12 supports the health of the nervous system and the development of red blood cells. It aids in the replication of the genetic code within each cell, and it plays a role in the processing of protein, fats, and carbohydrates.

Good food sources of vitamin B12: Clams, ham, herring, king crab, oysters (cooked), salmon, and tuna.

Vitamin C

Vitamin C prevents cell damage caused by free radicals. Your body's cells use oxygen to burn food for energy and to burn away germs and foreign chemicals, such as herbicides or pesticides. This process creates a tiny combustion in your cells that give off "sparks." These "sparks," chemically called free radicals, can start fires in other places, damaging cell membranes and destroying the fatty acids. Antioxidants, like vitamin C create your defense system against these free radicals. Your immune response depends on a number of vitamins and minerals, especially vitamin A, C, E, B2, B3, zinc, copper, manganese, and sulfur. Antioxidants increase the effectiveness of your nervous system, thereby increasing the power of your immune system. Vitamin C is also essential in the formation and maintenance of collagen, a protein that forms the basis for all of your connective tissue, and it helps maintain healthy skin, vision, and gums.

Good food sources of vitamin C: Broccoli, cantaloupe, kiwifruit, oranges, peppers, pineapple, pink grapefruit, and strawberries.

Vitamin D

Vitamin D functions as a pro-hormone by regulating the absorption and use of calcium and phosphorous. It aids in the formation of bones and teeth and plays an important role in healthy immune function. Vitamin D is also necessary for calcium absorption, which is why calcium supplements contain vitamin D.

Good food sources of vitamin D: Cereals (fortified), eggs, herring, milk (fortified), salmon, and sardines.

Vitamin E

Vitamin E protects the health and function of the nervous system and supports healthy skin.

Good food sources of vitamin E: Oils (safflower, soybean), spinach, sunflower seeds, wheat germ, and whole grains.

Vitamin K

Vitamin K is essential for blood clotting, and it plays an important role in bone formation and the regulation of blood calcium levels.

Good food sources of vitamin K: Broccoli (cooked), cauliflower, green leafy vegetables, liver, soybean oil and wheat bran.

Biotin

Biotin supports energy metabolism, and it maintains healthy skin, hair, and mucous membranes.

Good food sources of biotin: Barley, cauliflower, cereals (fortified), corn, egg yolks, milk, peanuts, soybeans, walnut and yeast.

Choline

Choline aids the production and transportation of fats from the liver and supports normal nerve and brain function.

Good food sources of choline: Whole eggs, liver, beef steak and soy.

Chromium

Chromium functions in the uptake of blood (glucose) or sugar levels into the cells and the regulation of blood sugar levels.

Good food sources of chromium: Brewer's yeast, broccoli, grape juice, and ham.

Copper

Copper helps to develop and maintain red blood cells, the cardiovascular system, and the skeletal system. Copper also aids the absorption and release of iron and the production of collagen, elastin, and melanin.

Good food sources of copper: Beans, cocoa powder, mushrooms, nuts, seeds, shellfish (especially cooked oysters), and whole grains.

Folic Acid

Folic acid regulates cell division and the transfer of inherited traits from one cell to another. Folic acid supports the gums, red blood cells, skin, gastrointestinal tract, and immune system.

Good food sources of folic acid: Asparagus, beans (navy and pinto), broccoli, cereals (fortified), lentils, okra, orange juice (fortified), and spinach.

Inositol

Inositol, a component of cell membranes, functions in nerve transmission and the regulation of certain enzymes. It is a lipotropic nutrient involved in the metabolism of fat.

Good food sources of inositol: Nuts, beans, wheat, cantaloupe and oranges.

Iodine

Iodine is component of thyroid hormones, which regulates metabolism, growth, reproduction, nerve, and muscle function. It is also involved in protein synthesis, the growth of skin and hair, and it's important in the use of oxygen by the cells.

Good food sources of iodine: Bread, iodized salt, lobster, marine fish, milk, oysters (cooked), and shrimp.

Iron

Iron acts as the oxygen-carrying component of blood, and it therefore determines how much oxygen reaches the body tissues, including the brain, muscles, heart, and liver. I do not recommend iron supplements to my male patients because iron can be formed into a ferris compound, one of the most prominent free radicals in the body. Free radicals weaken the body's immune system. Women, on the other hand, would benefit from taking iron due to blood loss associated with their menstrual cycles.

Good food sources of iron: Baked potatoes, beef, cereals (fortified), clams, pumpkin seeds, and soybeans.

Manganese

Manganese plays a role in connective tissue and bone formation, it supports reproduction and healthy brain function. As it is necessary for normal glucose metabolism, manganese also plays a role in energy production.

Good food sources of manganese: Cocoa powder, nuts, pineapple juice (canned), seeds, shellfish, tea, wheat bran, wheat germ, and whole grains.

Niacin

Niacin plays an important role in the release of energy from carbohydrates. Niacin aids in the breakdown of proteins and fats, the synthesis of fats, and the function of red blood cells.

Good food sources of niacin: Breads and cereals (fortified), chicken breast, tuna and veal.

PABA

PABA plays a role in B-vitamin metabolism as an enzyme cofactor.

Good food sources of PABA: Grains, greens (leafy), and rice (brown)

Pantothenic Acid

Pantothenic acid is converted to a substance called coenzyme A, an important catalyst in the breakdown of fats, proteins, and carbohydrates for energy. Pantothenic acid also plays a role in the production of fats, cholesterol, bile, vitamin D, red blood cells, adrenal gland hormones, and neurotransmitters.

Good food sources of pantothenic acid: Cereals (fortified), mushrooms, peanuts, salmon, and whole grains.

Phosphorus

Phosphorus is essential for healthy bones, teeth, soft tissues, and cell membranes. Phosphorus helps maintain the pH balance in the blood, and it also helps to activate the B vitamins.

Good food sources of phosphorus: Beef (extra-lean), cheese, chicken breast, halibut, lima beans, milk (fat-free), oatmeal (fortified), salmon, and yogurt (fat-free).

Potassium

Potassium plays a role in muscle contraction and relaxation, nerve conduction, regulation of the heartbeat, production of energy, and the synthesis of nucleic acids and proteins.

Good food sources of potassium: Apricots (dried), bananas, broccoli, coconut, carrots, and cucumbers.

You should not take all of these nutrients separately. I recommend that you take a (good) multiple vitamin daily. I don't recommend sugar-coated "one-a-day" type vitamins or cheap vitamins available at large discount chains. I recommend that you go to a health food or specific vitamin store to purchase vitamins. When it comes to vitamins, you will find that the old adage "you get what you pay for" is true. What good is it for any patient to take a vitamin that their body does not absorb? When I was in radiology class at chiropractic college, the instructor placed an x-ray of a person's midsection on the overhead. A small white dot was visible, and the instructor asked the class what it was. No one in the class knew, and he told them it was a sugar-coated vitamin in the large intestine that the body was unable to break down. What goes in doesn't always get absorbed, and it may come out.

Caffeine

I strongly recommend a low caffeine intake. Even when drinking decaf coffee or soda, you will be ingesting a small amount of caffeine, usually up to 5 mg. Caffeine impairs motor function (muscle function). It produces a let-down effect, resulting in fatigue and depression. It decreases immune function, resulting in a decreased resistance to infection. Caffeine also causes nervousness, muscle tension, irritability, heart palpitation, rapid breath, and shortness of breath. Ingesting large amounts of caffeine can cause restless leg syndrome, a condition where a person's legs will jump at night as he is about to go to sleep. Hyperactivity and insomnia are common in children who consume many caffeinated drinks. Caffeine certainly increases alertness, but this can be dangerous, because it is an artificial stimulant. Caffeine only masks fatigue.

Caffeine has been shown to cause cancer of the pancreas, one of the deadliest forms of cancer. Researchers at Harvard University state that coffee drinkers in the U.S. are twice as likely to develop pancreatic cancer. One to two cups of coffee per day doubles the risk of pancreatic cancer, and three or more triples it. Bladder cancer is also more prevalent among coffee and cola drinkers. Caffeine causes hyperacidity in the stomach. Hyperacidity is what causes the burning sensation reported by ulcer patients, and research shows that coffee drinkers have a 72% chance of developing ulcers. Caffeine allows for an increase of free fatty acids, causing an increase of blood fats and cholesterol, two factors associated with heart disease.

Consumers of caffeine greatly increase their chances of having a heart attack. When consuming up to 5 cups of coffee per day, the risk of a heart attack increases 60%, and this risk jumps to 120% if more than 5 cups are consumed per day. Caffeine can also produce sensory disturbances, such as ringing in the ears and spots before the eyes. Caffeine destroys important vitamins in our bodies, particularly vitamin B1 (thiamin), a nutrient that is crucial to mental health and tranquility. Caffeine also blocks the absorption of iron, leading in many cases to anemia. Caffeine can cause reoccurring headaches, and headaches can also occur from caffeine withdrawal. I have observed a large number of women in their 20's and 30's who don't drink coffee, but they drink three to four cans of Diet Mountain Dew per day. Mountain Dew and similar sodas contain the highest amounts of caffeine. "Jolt" even guarantees to give you a rush because of the amount of caffeine it contains. Finally, caffeine, causing lumps and nodules, predisposes women to fibrocystic breast disease. Caffeine has also been shown to increase the risk of breast cancer.

Nicotine

Nicotine is extremely addicting and very toxic to the brain. How do you quit smoking? I honestly do not have the answer since I have never smoked. The best method that I have gleened from others is "cold turkey", although nicotine patches, pills, and gum have worked for others. Whatever works for you is probably the best adage. If you are serious about getting well and staying well, you **must** quit smoking.

Sugar/Aspartame

Sugar, in large quantities, weakens the enzymes that metabolize essential fatty acids. It also adversely affects the efficiency of copper and the B vitamins. Sugar increases the amounts of magnesium and other important minerals excreted in the urine. It causes mood swings and fatigue. I recommend that you read two books concerning sugar: *Potatoes Not Prozac* by Kathleen DesMaisons, Ph.D. and *Sugar Blues* by William Dufty. These books are exceptional in explaining the adverse affects of sugar on the body.

Products like Nutrasweet, Equal, and Spoonful are actually aspartame, and when the temperature of aspartame exceeds 86 degrees Fahrenheit, the wood alcohol in aspartame turns to formaldehyde, then to formic acid, which in turn causes metabolic acidosis. Aspartame has been shown to cause fibromyalgia-like symptoms such as muscle spasms, shooting pains, numbness in the legs, cramps, dizziness, headaches, tinnitus, or ringing in the ears, joint pain, depression, anxiety, slurred speech, blurred vision, and memory loss. Unfortunately, I have seen many patients in my practice downing anywhere from six to twelve cans of diet soda per day. When I tell them what aspartame does to their nervous systems, many of them cut back or eliminate aspartame altogether.

Protein

I recommend a higher protein, lower fat diet to my patients because the chemicals that allow your nerve cells to communicate (neurotransmitters) are made up of amino acids. Your body breaks down proteins into amino acids. Lean meat, fish, lentils, fat-free dairy products, and nuts, especially almonds, are very high in protein. Almonds are the "kings of nuts" because they contain higher amounts of protein, vitamins, and fiber than other nuts. At breakfast, I recommend fresh fruit and/or juice. At lunch, I recommend a protein, any vegetable except corn, peas, and winter squash, and a small amount of carbohydrates (bread, rice, pasta or potato). At dinner, I do not recommend any carbohydrates, only a protein and a vegetable. Good choices for dinner would be a grilled chicken filet on top of a salad or a lean steak smothered in mushrooms with green beans and a salad. Many companies like Boca and Nature's Touch now produce vegetarian hamburger and chicken which are excellent sources of lowfat soy protein. You can use your imagination to come up with just about any meal plan you like.

Alcohol

I only recommend one to two alcoholic drinks per week, and I do not recommend binge drinking (consuming over five alcoholic drinks at one time). Alcohol adversely affects your brain, especially the cerebellum. When a person is pulled over by the police on suspicion of DUI (Driving Under the Influence), the policeman will ask the driver to touch his nose with his finger and walk in a straight line, and the policeman will check for nystagmus (eye bouncing). These are all cerebellar tests. The police perform these tests to determine the function of the brain, and I use many of these neurological tests in my office. When I was younger, I would joke that I was losing brain cells as a result of drinking too much alcohol. Believe me, folks, it is no joke. Alcohol is toxic to the neuron, or nerve cell, and repeated use will cause brain dysfunction. The book *Change your Brain - Change your Life* by David Amen, M.D. illustrates what excess alcohol, caffeine, and nicotine will do to the brain.

Detoxification

One of the treatments I utilize with patients is detoxification. Detoxification is very important for all people, but it is especially important for patients who suffer from chronic conditions like fibromyalgia and vertigo. We live in a toxic environment, and we have many refined additives in our food supply, including artificial preservatives, flavorings, colorings, and conditioners. Because of these artificial substances, agricultural antibiotics, and poor diets, many people are predisposed to internal pollution. Internal pollution occurs when the helpful bacteria in the intestinal tract are overcome by the unhelpful bacteria. This allows the body to become toxic. Internal pollution can also occur if a person smokes, consumes large quantities of alcohol, or consumes large quantities of caffeinated beverages. Detoxification can prevent a syndrome known as "leaky gut syndrome," a syndrome I first heard about from Jeffery Bland, Ph.D. "Leaky gut syndrome" occurs when toxins leak through the large intestine and flow into the liver. Toxins then leave the liver and pollute fat and brain tissues. When the liver is unable to detoxify, the stored toxins will circulate in the blood and contribute to a downward spiral of health. When our bodies are overloaded with toxic substances, we may experience pain, fatigue, mood swings, gastrointestinal irregularities, and flu-like symptoms. Extreme toxic overload may also contribute to more serious conditions such as autoimmune disease, inflammatory and rheumatoid arthritis, myastinia gravis, Alzheimer's disease, and Parkinson's disease. This has been documented clinically and in research. Metagenics is a company that produces some of the best prodcuts for detoxification in the country. I use their products exclusively in my offices.

Another great method of detoxifying your body is to purchase a home juicer. I strongly feel that anyone with a chronic health condition should be consuming fresh fruit and vegetable juices. Bottled or canned juices are <u>not</u> the answer. They contain unhealthy additives and lose much of their vitamins and minerals during the process of bottling or canning.

If you truly want to invest in your health, buy a juicer and USE IT! A juicer will not do you any good if it sits in the kitchen cabinet. Try consuming juices for an entire day. Fresh fruit juice in the morning to early afternoon and fresh vegetable juice from late afternoon to evening. Drink as much as you like. I guarantee that your well-being and energy level will improve.

Consume juice in place of a meal. Pick a meal (breakfast, lunch, or dinner) and consume fresh juice instead. Would you like to lose weight? Forget Slim Fast and drink juice! You can follow the Slim Fast meal plan but drink fresh juice instead of the can of Slim Fast.

Elimination Diet/Food Allergies

I also use an elimination diet to treat patients with food allergies. Headaches, muscle and joint pain, fatigue, irritability, depression, mental confusion, gastrointestinal irregularities, cardiovascular irregularities, flu-like symptoms, sneezing, and coughing may all be symptoms of food allergies. Many people have allergies to specific foods, including dairy, wheat, and processed meat. To determine if the patient has a food allergy, I instruct him/her to eliminate one of the following three groups for one week. If the symptoms abate, I know that the patient has a food allergy to that food group.

1. Eliminate dairy products, such as milk, cheese, and ice cream. (Note: Varying amounts of natural, unsweetened, live-culture yogurt may be tolerated by some individuals.)

2. Eliminate gluten. Avoid any food that contains wheat, spelt, kamut, oats, rye, barley, amaranth, quinoa, or malts. This is the most difficult part of the diet, but also the most important. Unfortunately, gluten is contained in many common foods, such as bread, crackers, pasta, and cereals. Products made from rice, corn, buckwheat, potato, tapioca, and arrowroot flours may be used as desired by most individuals.

3. Avoid red meats, such as beef, pork, or veal. Chicken, turkey, lamb, and cold-water fish, such as salmon, mackerel, and halibut, are acceptable if you are not allergic to these foods. Select from free-range meats whenever possible.

When following the elimination diet, patients should drink at least two quarts of water, preferably filtered water, daily. They should avoid all alcohol-containing products, including beer, wine, liquor, and over-the-counter products that contain alcohol. Also, they should avoid all caffeine-containing beverages, including coffee, caffeinated tea, and soda. Coffee substitutes from gluten-containing grains and decaffeinated coffee should also be avoided. I instruct patients to read labels carefully, as over-the-counter medications may contain alcohol or caffeine.

Chapter 12:
Prayer

"With God, All things Are Possible."
-Matthew 19:26

The cover of the November 10th, 2003 *Newsweek* reads: "God & Health: Is Religion Good Medicine? Why Science Is Starting To Believe."

Prayer is power. I consider myself a Christian and would be remiss if I did not include prayer as a dynamic healing potential. A patient handed me the following article entitled "Prayer is Power," written by Alexis Carrel, M.D. I don't know where the patient obtained this article, but I have it in my office and pull it out of my letterbox many times during the week.

"Prayer is Power"

Prayer is not only worship; it is also an invisible emanation of man's worshipping spirit, the most powerful form of energy that one can generate. The influence of prayer on the human mind and body is as demonstrable as that of secreting glands. Its results can be measured in terms of increased physical buoyancy, greater intellectual vigor, moral stamina, and a deeper understanding of the realities underlying human relationships.

If you make a habit of sincere prayer, your life will be very noticeably and profoundly altered. Prayer stamps with its indelible mark on our actions and demeanor. A tranquility of bearing and a facial and bodily repose are observed in those whose inner lives are thus enriched. Within the depths of consciousness, a flame kindles. And a man sees himself. He discovers his selfishness, his silly pride, his fears, his greed, his blunders. He develops a sense of moral obligation, intellectual humility. Thus begins a journey of the soul toward the realm of grace.

Prayer is a force as real as terrestrial gravity. As a physician, I have seen men, after all other therapy had failed, lifted out of disease and melancholy by the serene effort of prayer. It is the only power in the world that seems to overcome the so-called "laws of nature"; the occasions on which prayer has dramatically done this have been termed "miracles." But a constant, quieter miracle takes place hourly in the hearts of men and women who have discovered that prayer supplies them with a steady flow of sustaining power in their daily lives.

Too many people regard prayer as a formalized routine of words, a refuge for weaklings, or a childish petition for material things. We sadly undervalue prayer when we conceive it in these terms, just as we should underestimate rain by describing it as something that fills the birdbath in our garden. Properly understood, prayer is a mature activity indispensable to the fullest development of personality - the ultimate integration of man's highest faculties. Only in prayer do we achieve that complete and harmonious assembly of body, mind and spirit that gives the frail human reed its unshakable strength.

The words "ask and it shall be given to you" have been verified by the experience of humanity. True, prayer may not restore the dead child to life or bring relief from physical pain, but prayer, like radium, is a source of luminous, self-generating energy.

How does prayer fortify us with so much dynamic power? To answer this question admittedly outside the jurisdiction of science, I must point out that all prayers have one thing in common. The triumphant hosannas of a great oratorio and the humble supplication of an Iroquois hunter begging for luck in the chase demonstrate the same truth: human beings seek to augment their finite energy by addressing themselves to the infinite source of all energy. When we pray, we link ourselves with the inexhaustible motive power that spins the universe. We ask that a part of this power be apportioned to our needs. Even in asking, our human deficiencies are filled and we arise strengthened and repaired.

But we must never summon God merely for the gratification of our whims. We derive the most power from prayer when we use it not as a petition, but as a supplication that we may become more like him. Prayer should be regarded as practice of the presence of God. An old peasant was seated alone in the last pew of the village church. "What are you waiting for?" he was asked, and he answered, "I am looking at Him and He is looking at me." Man prays not only that God should remember him, but also that he should remember God.

How can prayer be defined? Prayer is the effort of man to reach God, to commune with an invisible being, creator of all things, supreme wisdom, truth, beauty, and strength, father and redeemer of each man. This goal of prayer always remains hidden to intelligence. For both language and thought fail when we attempt to describe God.

We do know that whenever we address God in fervent prayer, we change both soul and body for the better. It could not happen that any man or woman could pray for a single moment without some good result. "No man ever prayed," said Emerson, "without something."

One can pray everywhere. In the streets, the subway, the office, the shop, the school, as well as in the solitude of one's room, or among the crowd in a church. There is no prescribed posture, time or place.

"Think of God more often than you breathe," said Epictetus the Stoic. In order to really mold personality, prayer must become a habit. It is meaningless to pray in the morning and to live like a barbarian the remainder of the day. True prayer is a way of life; the truest life is literally a way of prayer.

The best prayers are like the improvisations of gifted lovers, always about the same thing, but never twice the same. We cannot all be as creative in prayer as Saint Theresa or Bernard of Clairvaux, both of whom poured their adoration into words of mystical beauty. Fortunately, we do not need their eloquence; our slightest impulse to pray is recognized by God. Even if we are pitifully dumb or if our tongues are overlaid with vanity or deceit, our meager syllables of praise are acceptable to Him, and He showers us with strengthening manifestations of His love.

Today, as never before, prayer is a blinding necessity in the lives of men and nations. The lack of emphasis on the religious sense has brought the world to the edge of destruction. Our deepest source of power and perfection has been left miserably undeveloped. Prayer, the basic exercise of the spirit, must be made strong enough to assert itself once more. For if the power of prayer is again released and used in the lives of common men and women, if the spirit declares its aims clearly and boldly, there is yet hope that our prayers for a better world will be answered.

- Alexis Carrel, M.D.

"We will either find a way, or we will make one."
                                    - Hannibal, 210 B.C.

Epilogue

As an old saying goes, you should begin at the beginning, end at the end, and put everything else in the middle. What do you do when the medications don't work? What do you do when your doctor tells you that he has tried everything and there is nothing more he can do for you? You don't have to suffer! There is a way out! After being in practice for over twenty years, my answer to you is to consult a board-certified chiropractic neurologist, specifically a Carrick-trained board-certified chiropractic neurologist. You can log on to the Chiropractic Neurology Board website at www.dacnb.org to find a chiropractic neurologist in your area. You have to be careful, as some of the chiropractic neurologists on the DACNB web site are not "Carrick-trained." You might want to call the doctor to quiz him about his knowledge of the Carrick examination and treatment modalities. There is an answer to your health condition. Never give up. Never quit.

To order CDs and/or consulting, or to
e-mail Dr. Johnson with a question go to:

www. askdrjohnson.com

Appendix I

Curriculum Vitae

I. Personal

Michael L. Johnson, D.C., D.A.C.N.B.(Diplomate
American Chiropractic Neurology Board)
Born: December 1, 1958, Escanaba, MI
Marital Status: Wife - Michele, and five children

II. Education

High School: A.D. Johnston High School, Bessemer, MI.
Graduated 1977
Undergraduate: Ferris State College, 1977-1980
Chiropractic College: Palmer College of Chiropractic,
Davenport, IA. Graduated March 18, 1983

III. Work Experience

Wood Chiropractic Clinic, Davenport, IA. Intern, 1981-
1983, Doctor of Chiropractic, March 1983 - June 1983
Johnson Chiropractic Office, Appleton, WI. September 1,
1983 - March 1999
Apple Chiropractic, Appleton, WI. April 1999 - present
Apple Medical Clinic, S.C., Appleton, WI. September 1,
1996 - present
Apple Medical Clinic, S.C., Green Bay, WI. February 17,
1998 - present
Apple Medical Clinic, S.C., Manitowoc, WI. May 4,
1999 - present

IV. Advanced Training and Professional Accomplishments

1980-1996 Gonstead Seminars, Mt. Horeb, WI.
Seventeen seminars at seventeen hours each (289 hours).

1980-1987   Gonstead Methodology, Davenport, IA.
Thirteen seminars at twelve hours each (156 hours).

1983   Parker Seminar, Chicago, IL. (18 hours)

1983-1987 Chiropractic Management Services (CMS),
various cities. (180 hours).

1985 Impairment Rating Seminar, National College of
Chiropractic, Chicago, IL. (15 hours)

1985 Sports Injuries Seminar, National College of
Chiropractic, Appleton, WI.   (96 hours).

1985-1991   Renaissance Seminars. various cities. (120
hours)

1986   Management by Statistics, Chicago, IL. (60 hours).

1986 Activator Seminars, Minneapolis, MN. (18 hours)

1988-1990   Applied Spinal Biomechanical Engineering
(A.S.B.E.), Chicago, IL.   (192 hours).

1990   Orthopedic Modules, National College of
Chiropractic, Chicago, IL (36 hours)

1988-1990 Sigafoose Seminars, various cities. (84
hours).

1989-1990   Nikitow Seminars Various cities. (60 hours)
1990   Neurology Modules, National College of
Chiropractic, Chicago, IL (36 hours).

1990   Pettibon Seminars, St. Cloud, MN. (15 hours)

1990 Kale Upper Cervical Specific, Chicago, IL. (12 hours).

1990-1996   N.E.T. Seminars, San Francisco, CA. (48 hours).

1990   Total Body Modification (TBM), Seattle, WA. (12 hours).

1990-1996   Chiropractic Biophysics, various cities. (68 hours).

1992   Minnesota Chiropractic Association, Northwestern College of Chiropractic, Nubbeaoikusm NB (20 hours).

1993   Schofield Personal & Professional Training, Phoenix, AZ (252 hours).

1994   Acupuncture Certification Course, National College of Chiropractic, Chicago, IL. and Davenport, IA (120 hours). Certified December 18, 1994.

1995   Cervical Spine Trauma and Rehabilitation, Chicago, IL and Clearwater, FL. (24 hours). Recertification in impairment rating.

1995 Mally Extremity Seminar. (48 hours). Certified June 1995 in extremity adjusting and carpal tunnel syndrome.

1996 Cervical Spine Trauma and Rehabilitation, Chicago, IL. (12 hours).

1996-present MD/DC Practice, various cities. (90 hours).

1997 Biokinetics Seminar, Chicago, IL. (12 hours).

1998 Cummings Seminars, Rochester, NY. (40 hours).

1997-present Chiropractic Neurology, Dr. Frederick Carrick, Parker College of Chiropractic, Dallas, TX., (750 hours).

2000 Second Opinion Consult Seminars, National College of Health Sciences, Chicago, IL (72 hours).

V. **Memberships and Associations**
American Chiropractic Association
ACA Council on Neurology
United Chiropractors of Wisconsin
1983 - National Board of Chiropractic Examiners
1983 - Gonstead Clinical Studies Society
1986 - ACA Council on Sports Injuries and Physical Fitness
1988 - American Academy of Clinical Applied Spinal Biomechanical Engineering

VI. **Awards**
1984 National Gonstead Research Society - Advancement in chiropractic research
1987 Foundation for the Advancement of Chiropractic Tenets and Science
1988 Federation of Chiropractic Education and Research - Advancement of chiropractic education and research
1994 Certified in Acupuncture
1999 Board Eligible Chiropractic Neurologist
2002 Board Certified Chiropractic Neurologist

Appendix II

The following references were provided to us by Dr. Carrick while attending the neurology modules in Dallas, TX.

Auditory Stimulation References

1. Huckins, 7S.C.; Turner, C.W.; Doherty, K.A.; Fonte, M.M.; Szeverenyi, N.M. functionalmagnetic resonance imaging measures of blood flow patterns in the human auditory cortex in response to sound. J-Speech-Lang-Hear-Res. 1998 Jun; 41(3): 538-48; ISSN: 1092-4388. UNITED STATES.

2. Ison, J. R.; Agrawal, P.; Pak, J.; Vaugh, W.J. Changes in temporal acuity with age and with hearing impairment in the mouse: a study of the acoustic startle reflex and its inhibition by brief decrements in noise level. J-Acoust-Soc-Am. 1998 Sep; 104(3 Pt 1): 1696-704: 0001-4966. UNITED STATES.

3. Britten, K.H.; Newsome, W.T. Tuning bandwidths for near-threshold stimuli in area MT. J-Neurophysiol. 1998 Aug; 80(2): 762-70; ISSN: 0022-3077.UNITED STATES.

4. Hillyard, S.A.; Tener Salejarvi, W.A.; Munte, T.F. Temporal dynamics of early perceptual processing. Curr-Opin-Neurobiol. 1998 Apr; 8(2): 202-10; ISSN 0959-4388. England.

5. Belin, P.; McAdams, S.; Smith, B.; Savel, S.; Thivard, L.; Samson, S.; Samson, Y. The functional anatomy of sound intensity discrimination. J-Neurosci. 1998 Aug 15;18(16): 6388-94; ISSN: 0270-6474. UNITED STATES.

6. Esser, K.H.; Condon, C.J.; Suga, N.; Kanwal, J.S. Syntax processing by auditory cortical neurons in the FM-FM area of the mustached bat Pternonotus pernellii. Proc-Natl-Acad-Sci-U-S-A. 1997 Dec 9; 94(25): 14019-24; ISSN: 007-8424. UNITED STATES.

7. Hendler, T.; Squires, N.K.; Moore, J.K.; Coyle, P. K. Auditory evoked potentials in multiple sclerosis: correlation with magnetic resonance imaging. J-Basic-Clin-Physiol-Pharmacol. 1996: 7(3):

245-78; ISSN: 0334-1534. England.

8. Harrington, D.L.; Haaland, K.Y.; Knight R.T. Cortical networks underlying mechanisms of time perception. J-Neurosci. 1998 Feb 1; 18(3): 1085-95; ISSN: 0270-6474. UNITED STATES.

9. Alden, J. D.; Harrison D.W.; Snyder K.A.; Everhart, D.E. Age differences in intention to left and right hemispace using a dichotic listening paradigm. Neuropsychiatry-Neuropsychol-Behav-Neurol. 1997 Oct; 10(4): 239-42; ISSN: 0894-878X. UNITED STATES.

10. Duan, M.L.; Canlon, B. Differences in forward masking after a temporary and a permanent noise-induces hearing loss. Audion-Neurootol. 1996 Nov; 1(6): 238-38; ISSN: 1420-3030. SWITZER-LAND.

11. Burkark, R.; Palmer, A.R. Response of chopper units in the ventral cochlear nucleus of the anaesthetised guinea pig to clicks-in-noise and click trains. Hear-Res. 1997 Aug; 110(1-2): 234-50; ISSN: 0378-5955. NETHERLANDS.

12. Berrebi, A.S.; Spiou, G.A. PEP-19 immunoreactivity in the cochlear nucleus and superior olive of the cat. Neuroscience. 1998 Mar; 83(2): 535-54; ISSN: 0306-4522. UNITED STATES.

13. Arslan, E.; Turrini, M.; Lupi, G.; Genovese, E: Orzan, E. Hearing threshold assessment with auditory brainstem response (ABR and ElectroCochleoGraphy (ECochG) in uncooperative children. Scand-Audio-Suppl. 1997; 46: 32-7; ISSN: 0107-8593. DEN-MARK.

14. Carson, S.R.; Katsanis, J.; Iacono, W.G.; McGue, M. Emotional modulation of the startle reflex in twins: preliminary findings. Biol-Psychol. 1997 Oct 10; 46(3): 235-46; ISSN: 0301-0511. NETHER-LANDS.

15. Braveman, I.; Jaber, L.; Levi, H.; Adelman, C.; Arons, K.S.; Fischel Ghodsian, N.; Shohat, M.; Elidan, J. Audiovestibular findings in patients with deafness caused by a mitochondrial susceptibility mutation and precipitated by an inherited nuclear mutation or aminoglycosides. Arch-Otolaryngol-Head-Neck-Surg. 1996 Sep; 122(9): 1001-4; ISSN: 0886-4470. UNITED STATES.

16. Bertoli, S.; Probst, R. The role of transient-evoked otoacoustic emission testing in the evaluation of elderly persons. Ear-Hear. 1997 Aug; 18(4): 286-93; ISSN: 0196-0202. UNITED STATES.

17. Blumenthal, T.D.; Schicatano, E.J.; Chapman, J.G.; Norris, C.M.; Ergenzinger, ER Jr. Prepulse effects on magnitude estimation of startle-eliciting stimuli and startle responses. Percept-Psychophys. 1996 Jan; 58(1): 73-80; ISSN: 0031-5117. UNITED STATES.

18. Ottaviani, F.; Di Girolame, S.; Briglia, G.; De Rossi, G.; Di Giuda, D.; Di Nardo, W. Tonotopic organization of human auditory cortex analyzed by SPET. Audiology. 1997 Sept. 36(5); 241-8; ISSN: 0020-6091

19. Grady, C. L.; Van Meter, J.W.; Maisog, J.M.; Pietrini, P.; Krasuski, J.; Rauschecker, J.P. Attention-related modulation of activity in primary and secondary auditory cortex. Neuroreport. 1997 Jul. 28; 8(11): 2511-6 ISSN: 0959-4965

20. Lechevalier, B. (Perception of musical sounds: contributions of positron emission tomography). La perception des sons musicaux: apports de la camera a position. Bull-Acad-Natl-Med-Med. 1997 Jun; 181(6): 1191-9; discussion 1199-200; ISSN: 0001-4079.

21. Ofemann, J.G.; Neil, J.M.; MacLeod, A.M.; Silbergeld, D.L.; Dacey, RG Jr.; Petersen, S.E.; Raichle, M.E. Increased functional vascular response in the region of the glioma. J-Cereb-Blood-Flow-

Metab. 1998 Feb; 18(20): 148-53; ISSN: 0271-678X.

22. Schumacher,. E.H.; Lauber, E.; Awh, E.; Jonides, J.; Smith, E.E.; Koeppe, R.A. PET evidence for an amodal verbal working memory system. Neuroimage. 1996 Apr; 3(20): 79-88; ISSN: 1053-8119.

Big Letter Stimulation References

1. Fink, G.R.; Halligan, P.W.; Marshall, J. C.; Frith, C.D.; Frackowiak, R. S.; Dolan, R. J. Neural mechanism involved in the processing of global and local aspects of hierarchically organized visual stimuli. Brain. 1997 Oct.; 120(Pt 10): 1779-91; ISSN 0006-8950.

2. Burgund, E. D.; Marsolek, C. J. Letter-case-specific priming in the right cerebral hemisphere with a form-specific perceptual identification task. Brain-Cogn. 1997 Nov; 35(2): 239-58; ISSN: 0278-2626.

3. Burguns, E. D.; Marsolek, C. J. Letter-case-specific priming in the right cerebral hemisphere with a form-specific perceptual identification task. Brain-Cogn. 1997 Nov; 35(2): 239-58; ISSN: 0278-2626. UNITED-STATES.

4. Fink, G. R.; Halligan, P. W.; Marshall, J. C.; Frith, C. D.; Frackowiak, R. S.; Dolan, R. J. Neural mechanisms involved in the processing of global and local aspect of hierarchically organized visual stimuli. Brain. 1997 Oct.; 120(Pt 10): 1779-91; ISSN: 0006-8950.ENGLAND.

Eye Exercise References

1. Bremmer, F.; Pouget, A.; Hoffman, K.P. Eye position encoding in the macaque posterior parietal cortex. Eur-J-Neurosci. 1998 Jan;

10(1): 153-60; ISSN: 0953-816X. FRANCE.

2. TI: Eye movements in normal subjects induces by vibratory acti-vation of neck muscle proprioceptors.
AU: Han-Y; Lennerstrand-G
AD: Department of Ophthalmology, Karolinske Institute, Huddinge University Hospital, Sweden.
SO: Acta-Ophthalmol-Scand. 1995 Oct; 73(5): 414-6
ISSN: 1395-3907

3. Dejardin, S.; Dubois, S.; Bodart, J.M.; Schiltz, C.; Delinte, A.; Michel C,; Roucoux, A; Crommelinck, M. PET study of human voluntary saccadic eye movements in darkness: effect of task repe-tition on the activation pattern. EUR-J-Neurosci. 1998 Jul; 10(7): 2328-36; ISSN: 0953-816X. FRANCE.

Face References

1. Dolan, R.J.; Fletcher, P.; Morris, J.; Kapur, N.; Deakin, J.F.; Frith, C.D. Neural activation during covert processing of positive emotional facial expressions. Neuroimage. 1996 Dec; 4(3 Pt 1): 194-200; ISSN: 1053-8119. UNITED STATES.

2. Gabrieli, J.D.; Poldrack, R.A.; Desmond, J.E. The role of left prefrontal cortex in language and memory. Proc-Natl-Acad-Sci-U-S-A. 1998 Feb 3; 95(3): 906-12; ISSN: 0027-8424. UNITED STATES.

Hand Exercise References

1. Decety, J.; Grezes, J.; Costes, N.; Perani, D.; Jeannerod, M.; Procky, E.; Grassl, F.; Fazio, F. Brain activity during observation of actions. Influence of action content and subject's strategy. Brain 1997 Oct.; 120(Pt 10): 1763-77; ISSN: 0006-8950.

2. Davey, N. J.; Rawlinson, S. R.; Maskill, D. W.; Ellaway, P. H. Facilitation of a hand muscle response to stimulation of the motor cortex preceding a simple reaction task. Motor-Control. 1998 Jul; 2(3): 241-50; ISSN: 1087-1640. UNITED-STATES.

3. Chen, R; Yaseen, Z.; Cohen, L. G.; Hallett, Time course of corticospinal excitability in reaction time and self-paced movements. Ann-Neurol. 1998 Sept; 44(3): 317-25; ISSN: 0364-5134.UNITED-STATES.

4. Gitelman, D. R.; Alpert, N. M.; Kosslyn, S.; Daffner, K.; Scinto, L.; Thompson, W.; Mesulam, M. M. Functional imaging of human right hemispheric activation for exploratory movements. Ann-Neurol. 1996 Feb. 39(20): 17-9; ISSN: 036-513>UNITED-STATES.

5. Amunts, K.; Schlaug, G.; Schleicher, A.; Steinmetz, H; Dabringhaus, A.; Roland, P. E.; Zilles, K. Asymmetry in the human motor cortex and handedness. Neuroimage. 1996 Dec; 4(3 Pt 1): 216-22; ISSN: 1053-8119.UNITED-STATES.

Maze References

1. Pashek, G.V.; A case study of gesturally cued naming in aphasia: dominant versus nondominant hand training. J-Connun-Disord. 1997 Sept.; 30(5): 349-65; quiz 365-6; ISSN: 0021-9924.

2. Gillner, S.; Mallot, H. A. Navigation and acquisition of spatial-knowledge in a virtual maze. J-Cogn-Neurosci. 1998 Jul; 10(4): 445-63; ISSN: 0898-929X. UNITED-STATES.

Stroke References

1. Bernhardt, J.; Ellis, P.; Denisenko, S.; Hill, K. Changes in balance and locomotion measures during rehabilitation following

stroke. Physiother-Res-Int. 1998; 3(2): 109-22; ISSN: 1358-2267. ENGLAND.

2. Cruz martinez, A.; Munoz, J.; Palacios, F. The muscle inhibitory period by transcranial magnetic stimulation. Study in stroke patients. Electromyogr-Clin-Neurophysiol. 1998 Apr; 38(3): 189-92; ISSN: 0301-150X. BELGIUM.

3. Ballanyi, K.; lalley, P.M.; Hoch, B.; Richter, D.W. cAMP-dependent reversal of opioid-and prostaglandin-mediated depression of the isolated respiratory network in newborn rats. J-Physiol-Lond. 1997 Oct 1; 504(Pt 1): 127-34; ISSN: 0022-3751.ENGLAND.

4. Ahonen, J.P.; Jehkonen, M.; Dastibar, P.; Molnar, G.; Hakkinen, V. Cortical silent period evoked by transcranial magnetic stimulation in ischemic stroke. Electroencephalogr-Clin-Neurophysiol. 1998 Jun; 109(3): 224-9; ISSN: 0013-4694. IRELAND.

5. Crary, M.A.; Baldwin, B.O. Surface electromyographic characteristics of swallowing in dysphagia secondary to brainstem stroke. Dysphagia. 1997 Sep; 12(4): 180-7; ISSN: 0179-051X. UNITED-STATES.

6. Bandinelli, G.; Cencetti, S.; Buccheri, A.M.; Lagi, A. Noninvasive assessment of posterior cerebral artery stenosis inducing hemiplegia. Ann-Ital-Med-Int. 1997 Jan 12(1): 31-4; ISSN: 0393-9394. ITALY.

7. Kim, J.S.; Lee, J.H.; Choi, C. G. Pattern of lateral medullary infarction: vascular lesion-magnetic resonance imaging correlation of 34 cases. Stroke. 1998 Mar; 29(3): 645-52; ISSN: 0039-2499. UNITED-STATES.

8. Camuscu, H.; Dujovny, M.; Abd, el bary T.; Beristain, X.; Vinas,

F.C. Microanatomy of the perforators of the anterior communicating artery complex. Neurol-Res. 1997 Dec; 19(6): 577-87; ISSN: 0161-6412. ENGLAND.

9. Harber, E.S.; O'Sullivan, M.G.; Jayo, M.J.; Carlson, C.S. Cerebral infarction in two cynomolgus macaques (Macaca fascicularis) with hypernatremia. Vet-Pathol. 1996 Jul; 33(4): 431-4; ISSN: 0300-9858. UNITED-STATES.

10. Bruning, R.; Wu, R.H.; Diemling, M.; Porn, U.; Haberl, R.L.; Reiser, M. Diffusion measurements in the ischemic human brain with a steady-state sequence. Invest-Radiol. 1996 Nov; 31(11): 709-15; ISSN: 0020-9996. UNITED-STATES.

11. Butterworth, R.J.; Wassif, W. S.; Sherwood, R.A.; Gerges, A.; Poyser, K.H.; Garthwaite, J.; Peters, T.J.; Bath, P.M. Serum neuron-specific enolase, carnosinase, and their ratio is acute stroke. An enzymatic test for predicting outcome? Stroke. 1996 Nov; 27(11): 2064-8; ISSN: 0039-2499. UNITED STATES.

12. Kim, J.S.; Im, J.H.; Kwon, S.U.; Kang, J.H.; Lee, M.C. micrographia after thalamo-mesencephalic infarction: evidence of striatal dopaminergic hypofunction. Neurology. 1998 Aug; 51(2): 625-7; ISSN: 0028-3878. UNITED STATES.

13. Elger, B.; Hornberger, W.; Schwarz, M.; Seega, J.; MRI study on delayed ancrod therapy of focal cerebral ischaemia in rats. Eur-J-Pharmacol. 1997 Oct. 1; 336(1): 7-14; ISSN: 0014-2999. NETHERLANDS.

Visual Stimulation References

1. Chen, E.; Kato, T.; Zhu, H. H.; Strupp, J.; Ogawa, S; Ugurbil, K. Mapping of lateral geniculate nucleus activation during visual stimulation in human brain using firm. Magn-Reson-Med. 1998

Jan. 39(1): 89-96; ISSN: 0740-3194. UNITED-STATES.

2. Fransson, P.; Kruger, G; Merboldt, K. D.; Frahm, J. A. comparative FLASH and EPI study of repetitive and sustained visual activation. NMR-Biomed. 1997 Jun; 10(4-5): 204-7; ISSN: 0952-3480.ENGLAND.

3. Buchner, H.; Gobbele, R; Wagner, M.; Fuchs, M; Waberski, T. D.; Bechmann, R. Fast visual evoked potential input into human area V5. Neuroreport. 1997 Jul. 28; 8(11): 2419-22; ISSN: 0959-4965.ENGLAND.

4. Garacia Perez, M. A.; Sierra Vazquez, V. The optimal motion stimulus: comments on Watson and Turano (1995) [letter]. Vision-Res. 1998 Jun; 38(11): 1611-21; ISSN: 0042-6989. ENGLAND.

5. Jackson, S. R.; Husain, M. Visuomotor functions of the lateral pre-motor cortex. Curr-Opin-Neurobiol 1996 Dec; 6(6): 788-95; ISSN: 0959-1388.ENGLAND.

6. Epelboim, J.; Steinman, R. M.; Kowler, E.; Pizlo, Z.; Erkelens, C. J.; Collewijn, H. Gaze-shift dynamics in two kinds of sequential looking tasks. Vision-Res. 1997 Sep. 37(18): 2597-607; ISSN: 0042-6989.ENGLAND.

7. Furman, J. M.; Mendoza, J. C. Visual-vestibular interaction during off-vertical axis rotation. J-Vestib-Res. 1996 Mar;6(2): 93-103; ISSN: 0957-4271. UNITED-STATES.

8. Cornelius, C. P.; Altenmuller, E.; Ehrenfeld, M. The use of flash visual evoked potentials in the early diagnosis of suspected optic nerve lesions due to craniofacial trauma. J-Craniomaxillofac-Surg.1996 Feb; 24(1): 1-11; ISSN: 1010-5182. SCOTLAND.

9. TI: Egocentric visual target position and velocity coding: role

of ocular muscle proprioception.
AU: Gauthier-GM; Vercher-JL; Blouin-J
AD: Laboratorie de Controles Sensorimoteurs, Universite de Provence, Marseille, France.
SO: Ann-Biomed-Eng. 1995 Jul-Aug; 23(4): 423-35
ISSN: 0090-6964

10. Johansson, G.; Ahlstrom, U. Visual bridging of empty gaps in the optic flow. Percept-Psychophys. 1198 Aug; 60(6): 915-25; ISSN: 0031-5117. UNITED-STATES.

Word Search/List References

1. Andreasen, N. C.; O'Leary, D. S.; Cizadlo, T.; Arndt, S.; Rezai, K.; Watking, G. L.: Ponto, L. L.; Hichwa, R. D. II. PET studies of memory: novel versus practiced free recall of word lists. Neuroimage. 1995 Dec.; 2(4): 296-305; ISSN: 1053-8119

2. Henriques, J. B.; Davidson, R. J.; Brain electrical asymmetries during cognitive task performance in depressed and nondepressed subjects. Biol-Psychiatry. 1997 Dec. 1; 42(11): 1039-50; ISSN: 0006-3223.

3. Paradiso, D.; Crespo Facoaao, B.; Andreasen, N. C.; O'Leary, D. S.; Watkins, L. G.; Boles Ponto, L.; Hichwa, R. D. Brain activity assessed with PET during recall of word lists and narratives. Neuroreport. 1997 Sept. 29: 8(14): 3091-6; ISSN: 0959-4965

4.Schiffer, F. Cognitive activity of right hemisphere: possible contributions to psychological function. Harv-Rev-Psychiatry. 1996 Sept; 4(3): 126-38: ISSN: 1067-3229.

Appendix III

Medications and Possible Side Effects

Dimenhydrinate
(Meclizine)

Prescribed for Nausea, vomiting, and dizziness associated with motion sickness.

Possible side effects: **Most common:** drowsiness. **Least common:** confusion, nervousness, excitement, restlessness, headache, sleeplessness (especially in children), tingling, heavy or weak hands, fainting, dizziness, tiredness, rapid heartbeat, low blood pressure, heart palpitations, blurred or double vision, appetite loss, nausea, vomiting, diarrhea, upset stomach, constipation, nightmares, rash, drug reaction, ringing or buzzing in the ears; dry mouth, nose, or throat; stuffy nose, wheezing, and increased chest phlegm, or chest tightness.

Tiagabine
(Neurontin)

Prescribed for partial seizure. (anticonvulsant)

Possible side effects: Side effects occur in 60% of all people who administered this drug. **Most common:** diarrhea, nausea, upset stomach, rash, and stomach pain. **Least common:** reduced white-blood cell counts, vomiting, bruising, gas, itching, dizziness, appetite loss, and liver function changes.

Celecoxib
(Celebrex)

Prescribed for osteoarthritis and rheumatoid arthritis, familial adenomatous polyposis.

Possible side effects: **Most common:** headaches. **Least common:** diarrhea, upset stomach, sinus irritation, and respiratory infection.

Rofecoxib
(Vioxx)
Prescribed for osteoarthritis, painful menstruation, and acute pain.

Possible side effects: **Most common:** People taking any NSAID can develop a group of symptoms known as the aspirin triad. This occurs in people with asthma. The symptoms may include runny nose with or without nasal polyps and severe, potentially fatal broncial spasm. People who have these symptoms must report to the emergency room immediately. **Least common:** rash, itching, unexplained weight gain, nausea, fatigue, yellowing of the skin, flu-like symptoms, lethargy, swelling, black stools, severe stomach pain, and persistent headache.

Mirtazapine
(Remeron)
Prescribed for depression, tremors, and panic disorder.

Possible side effects: **Most common:** tiredness, dizziness, dry mouth, constipation, increased appetite, weight gain, large increases in blood cholesterol or triglyceride levels, weakness, and flu symptoms. **Least common:** back pain, nausea, vomiting, muscle ache, abnormal dreaming or thinking, anxiety, agitation, confusion, tremors, itching, rash, breathing difficulties, and frequent urination.

Toprol XL
(Ultram)
Prescribed for mild to moderate pain.

Possible side effects: **Most common:** dizziness or fainting, nausea, constipation, headache, tiredness, vomiting, itching, weakness, sweating, upset stomach, dry mouth, and diarrhea. **Least common:** feeling unwell, warmth and flushing, nervousness, anxiety,

agitation, euphoria (feeling "high"), emotional instability, trouble sleeping, abdominal pain, appetite loss, gas, rash, visual disturbances, urinary difficulties, and symptoms of menopause.

Zithromax, Zocor, Zoloft, Zolpidem (Ambien)
Prescribed for insomnia, sedative.

Possible side effects: **Most common:** drowsiness, dizziness, and diarrhea. **Least common:** chest pain, fatigue, unusual dreams, memory loss, anxiety, nervousness, difficulty sleeping, appetite loss, vomiting, and runny nose.

Trazodone (Desyrel)
Prescribed for depression with or without anxiety, cocaine withdrawal, panic disorder, agoraphobia (fear of open spaces), and aggressive behavior.
Possible side effects: **Most common:** upset stomach, constipation, abdominal pains, a bad taste in the mouth, nausea, vomiting, diarrhea, palpitations, rapid heartbeat, rash, swelling of the arms, or legs, blood pressure changes, breathing difficulties, dizziness, anger, hostility, nightmares, vivid dreams, confusion, disorientation, loss of memory or concentration, drowsiness, fatigue, light headedness, difficulty sleeping, nervousness, excitement, headache, loss of coordination, tingling in the hands or feet, tremor of the hands or arms, ringing or buzzing in the ears, blurred vision, red, tired, and itchy eyes, stuffy nose, or sinuses, loss of sex drive, muscle ache and pain, appetite loss, weight gain or loss, increased sweating, clamminess, and feeling unwell. **Least common:** drug allergy, chest pain, heart attack, delusions, hallucinations, agitation, difficulty speaking, restlessness, numbness, weakness, seizures, increased sex drive, reverse ejaculation, impotence, missed or early

menstrual periods, gas, increased salivation, anemia, reduced levels of certain white blood cells, muscle twitches, blood in the urine, reduced appetite. Trazodone may cause elevations in levels of body enzymes, which are used to measure liver function.

Tricyclic Antidepressants, Amitriptyline
(Elavil)
Prescribed for depression with or without symptoms of anxiety or sleep disturbance, chronic pain due to migraine, tension headaches, diabetic disease, tic douloureux, cancer, herpes lesions, and arthritis, pathologic laughing or weeping caused by brain disease, bulimia, sleep apnea, peptic ulcer disease, cocaine withdrawal, panic disorder, eating disorder, premenstrual depression, and skin problems.

Possible side effects: **Most common:** sedation and anticholinergic effects including blurred vision, disorientation, confusion, hallucinations, muscle spasm or tremors, seizures or convulsions, dry mouth, constipation, especially in older adults, difficulty urinating, worsening glaucoma, and sensitivity to bright light. **Least common:** blood pressure changes, abnormal heart rate, heart attack, anxiety, restlessness, excitement, numbness and tingling in the extremities, poor coordination, rash, itching, fluid retention, fever, allergy, changes in blood composition, nausea, vomiting, appetite loss, upset stomach, diarrhea, enlargement of the breasts in men and women, changes in sex drive, and blood-sugar changes.

Flexeril
(Cyclobenzaprine)
Prescribed for serious muscle spasm and acute muscle pain, also used to treat fibrositis (muscular rheumatism).

Possible side effects: **Most common:** dry mouth, drowsiness, and dizziness. **Least common:** muscle weakness, fatigue, nausea,

constipation, upset stomach, unpleasant taste, blurred vision, headache, nervousness, and confusion.

Soma
(Carisoprodol)
Prescribed for pain and discomfort associated with sprain, strain, and back problems.

Possible side effects: **Most common:** drowsiness. **Least common:** rapid heartbeat, dizziness or light headedness, fainting, depression, large hive-like swellings on the face, eyelids, mouth, lips, or tongue, breathing difficulties, chest tightness or wheezing, allergic fever, stinging or burning eyes, headache, unusual stimulation, trembling, upset stomach or abdominal cramps, hiccups, and nausea or vomiting.

Xanax
(Alprazolam)
Prescribed for anxiety, tension, fatigue, and agitation, also prescribed for irritable bowel syndrome, panic attacks, depression, and premenstrual syndrome (PMS).

Possible side effects: **Most common:** mild drowsiness during the first few days of therapy. Weakness and confusion may occur, especially in seniors and in those who are sickly. **Least common:** depression, lethargy, disorientation, headache, inactivity, slurred speech, stupor, dizziness, tremors, constipation, dry mouth, nausea, inability to control urination, sexual difficulties, irregular menstrual cycle, changes in heart rhythm, low blood pressure, fluid retention, blurred or double vision, itching, rash, hiccups, nervousness, inability to fall asleep, and occasional liver dysfunction.

Klonopin
(Clonazepam)

Prescribed for petit mal and other seizure; also prescribed for panic attacks, periodic leg movements during sleep, speaking difficulty associated with Parkinson's disease, acute manic episodes, nerve pain, and schizophrenia.

Possible side effects: **Most common:** drowsiness, poor muscle control, and behavioral changes. **Least common:** rare side effects can occur in most parts of the body but most likely will affect the mental function, stomach and intestines, urinary function, blood, and liver.

Imitrex
(Triptan-Type Antimigraine Drugs)

Prescribed for migraine headaches.

Possible side effects: **Most common:** nausea, vomiting, dizziness, fainting, a feeling of ill health, drowsiness, and sedation, tingling in the hands, feet, chest, neck, jaw, or symptoms of throat tightness or heaviness, tiredness, and weakness. **Least common:** diminished sensitivity to stimulation, heart palpitations, chest pain or pressure, sweating, and muscle aches.

Prozac
(Fluoxetine)

Prescribed for depression, bulimic binge-eating and vomiting, and obsessive-compulsive disorder, also prescribed for obesity, alcoholism, anorexia, attention-deficit hyperactivity disorder, bipolar affective disorder, borderline personality disorder, cataplexy and carcolepsy, kleptomania, migraine, chronic daily headache, tension headaches, post-traumatic stress disorder, schizophrenia, Tourette's syndrome, dyskinetic side effects of levodopa, and social phobias.

Possible side effects: **Most common:** headache, anxiety, nervousness, sleeplessness, drowsiness, tiredness, weakness, tremors, sweating, dizziness, light-headedness, dry mouth, upset or irritated stomach, appetite loss, nausea, vomiting, diarrhea, gas, rash, and itching. **Least common:** changes in sex drive, abnormal ejaculation, impotence, abnormal dreams, difficulty concentrating, increased appetite, acne, hair loss, dry skin, chest pain, allergy, runny nose, bronchitis, abnormal heart rhythms, bleeding, blood pressure changes, dizziness, or fainting when rising suddenly from a sitting position, bone pain, bursitis, twitching, breast pain, fibrocystic disease of the breast, cystitis, urinary pain, double vision, blood sugar, and low thyroid activity.

Zoloft
(Sertraline)
Prescribed for depression, also prescribed for obsessive compulsive disorder.
Possible side effects: **Most common:** dry mouth, headache, dizziness, tremors, nausea, diarrhea or loose stools, sleeplessness, tiredness, male sexual dysfunction or abnormal ejaculation, female sexual dysfunction, feeling ill, excessive sweating, constipation, upset stomach, and agitation. **Least common:** heart palpitations, chest pain, nervousness, anxiety, tingling or numbness in the hands or feet, twitching, muscle spasm, confusion, rash, muscle and joint ache, gas, appetite increase or decrease, menstrual disorders, sore throat, runny nose, yawning, changes in vision, ringing or buzzing in the ears, frequent urination, fever, back pain, chills, confusion, reduced skin sensation, rash, nightmares, depersonalization, weight gain, vomiting, and changes in sense of taste.

Antivert
(Dimenhydrinate)
Prescribed for nausea, vomiting, and dizziness associated with motion sickness.

Possible side effects: **Most common:** drowsiness. **Least common:** confusion, nervousness, excitement, restlessness, headache, sleeplessness, especially in children, tingling, heavy or weak hands, fainting, dizziness, tiredness, rapid heartbeat, low blood pressure, painful urination, increased sensitivity to the sun, appetite loss, nausea, vomiting, diarrhea, upset stomach, constipation, nightmares, rash, drug reaction, ringing or buzzing in the ears, dry mouth, nose, or throat, stuffy nose, wheezing, and increased chest phlegm or chest tightness.

Paxil
(Paroxetine)
Prescribed for depression, panic disorder, social anxiety, obsessive compulsive disorder, and post-traumatic stress, also prescribed for diabetic nerve disease, headache, and premature ejaculation.
Possible side effects: **Most common:** headache, weakness, sleep disturbances, dizziness, tremors, nausea, excessive sweating, weakness, dry mouth, decreased sex drive, abnormal ejaculation, blurred vision, and weight gain. **Least common:** flushing, pinpoint pupils, increased saliva, cold and clammy skin, dizziness when rising quickly from a seated position, blood pressure changes, swelling around the eyes and in the arms or legs, coldness in the hands or feet, fainting and dizziness, rapid heartbeat, weakness, loss of coordination, unusual walk, changes in the general level of activity, migraine, droopy eyelids, tingling in the hands or feet, acne, hair loss, dry skin, difficulty swallowing, gas, joint pain, muscle pain, cramps and weakness, aggressiveness, abnormal dreaming or thinking, memory loss, apathy, delusions, feelings of detachment, worsened depression, emotional instability, euphoria ("high

feeling"), hallucinations, neurosis, paranoia, suicide attempts, teeth grinding, menstrual cramps or pain, bleeding between periods, coughing, bronchospasm, nosebleed, breathing difficulties, conjunctivitis, double vision, difficulty accommodating to bright light, eye pain, earache, painful urination, facial swelling, frequent urination, nighttime urination, loss of urinary control, generalized swelling, not feeling well, and lymph swelling.

Dilantin
(Phenytoin)
Prescribed for epileptic seizure, also prescribed for prevention of seizure following neurosurgery in nonepileptics and for abnormal heart rhythm.

Possible side effects: **Most common:** rapid or unusual growth of the gums, slurred speech, mental confusion, nystagmus (rhythmic, uncontrolled movement of the eye), dizziness, insomnia, nervousness, uncontrollable twitching, double vision, tiredness, irritability, depression, tremors, headache. **Least common:** nausea, vomiting, diarrhea, constipation, fever, rash, balding, weight gain, numbness in the hands or feet, chest pain, water retention, sensitivity to bright light (especially sunlight), conjunctivitis (pink eye), joint pain and inflammation, and high blood sugar.

Lorazepam
(Diazepam)
Prescribed for anxiety, tension, fatigue, agitation, muscle spasm, and seizures, also prescribed for irritable bowel syndrome and panic attacks.

Possible side effects: **Most common:** mild drowsiness, weakness and confusion may occur. **Least common:** depression, lethargy, disorientation, headache, inactivity, slurred speech, stupor, dizzi

ness, tremors, constipation, dry mouth, nausea, inability to control urination, sexual difficulties, irregular menstrual cycle, changes in heart rhythm, low blood pressure, fluid retention, blurred or double vision, itching, rash, hiccups, nervousness, inability to fall asleep, and occasional liver dysfunction.

Naproxen
(Naproxen Sodium)

Prescribed for rheumatoid arthritis, osteoarthirtis, ankylosing spondylitis, mild to moderate pain, tendinitis, bursitis, gout, fever, sunburn, migraine, and menstrual pain and headache.

Possible side effects: **Most common:** diarrhea, nausea, vomiting, constipation, gas, stomach upset or irritation, and appetite loss, especially during the first few days of treatment. **Least common:** stomach ulcers, GI bleeding, hepatitis, gallbladder attacks, painful urination, poor kidney function, kidney inflammation, blood and protein in the urine, dizziness, fainting, nervousness, depression, hallucination, confusion, disorientation, tingling in the hands or feet, light-headedness, itching, increased sweating, dry nose and mouth, heart palpitations, chest pain, difficulty breathing, and muscle cramps.

Effexor
(Venlafaxine)

Prescribed for depression.

Possible side effects: **Most common:** blurred vision, tiredness, dry mouth, dizziness, sleeplessness, nervousness, tremors, weakness, sweating, nausea, constipation, appetite loss, vomiting, impotence, and abnormal ejaculation. **Least common:** changes in sense of taste, ringing in the ears, dilated pupils, high blood pressure, rapid heartbeat, anxiety, reduced sex drive, agitation, chills, yawning, and inability to experience orgasm.

Serzone
(Nefazodone)
Prescribed for depression.

Possible side effects: **Most common:** weakness, dry mouth, nausea, constipation, blurred or abnormal vision, tiredness, dizziness, light-headedness, confusion, upset stomach, increased appetite, cough, memory loss, tingling in the hands and feet, flushing or feelings of warmth, poor muscle coordination, and dizziness when rising from a seated position. **Least common:** low blood pressure, fever, chills, flu-like symptoms, joint pain, stiff neck, itching, rash, diarrhea, nausea, vomiting, thirst, sore throat, changes in sense of taste, ringing or buzzing in the ear, unusual dreams, poor coordination, tremors, muscle stiffness, reduced sex drive, urinary difficulties including infection, vaginitis, and breast pain.

Darvocet, Darvon
(Propoxyphene Hydrochloride)
Prescribed for mild to moderate pain.

Possible side effects: **Most common:** dizziness, sedation, nausea, and vomiting. **Least common:** constipation, stomach pain, rash, light-headedness, headache, weakness, euphoria, and minor visual disturbances. Taking propoxyphene hydrochloride over long periods of time and in very high doses has caused psychotic reactions and convulsions.

Depakote
(Valproic Acid)
Prescribed for petit mal and absence seizure and bipolar (manic-depressive) disorder, also prescribed for grand mal, myoclonic, and other seizures, prevention of fever convulsions in children, migraine, and anxiety or panic attacks.

Possible side effects: **Most common:** nausea, vomiting, indigestion, sedation or sleepiness, weakness, rash, emotional upset, depression, psychosis, aggression, hyperactive behavior, and changes in blood components. **Least common:** diarrhea, stomach cramps, constipation, increased or decreased appetite, headache, loss of eye-muscle control, drooping eyelids, double vision, spots before the eyes, loss of muscle control or coordination, and tremors.

Coumadin
(Warfarin)
Prescribed for blood clots or coagulation; also prescribed for reducing the risk of small cell carcinoma of the lung, recurrent heart attack or stroke, and transient ischemic attack (TIA).
Possible side effects: **Most common:** bleeding, which may occur with usual dosages and even when the results of blood tests used to monitor anticoagulant therapy are normal. **Least common:** abdominal cramps, nausea, vomiting, diarrhea, fever, anemia, adverse effects on blood components, hepatitis, jaundice, itching, rash, hair loss, sore throat or mouth, red or orange urine, painful or persistent erection, and purple toe syndrome.

Inderal
(Propranolol)
Prescribed for high blood pressure, angina pectoris, abnormal heart rhythm, prevention of second heart attack or migraine, tremors, aggressive behavior, side effects of antipsychotic drugs, acute panic, stage fright and other anxieties, and schizophrenia, also used to treat bleeding from the stomach or esophagus, and symptoms of hyperthyroidism.

Possible side effects: **Most common:** impotence. **Least common:** tiredness or weakness, slow heartbeat, heart failure, dizziness, breathing difficulties, bronchospasm, depression, confusion, anxiety, nervousness, emotional instability, cold hands and feet, constipation, sweating, urinary difficulties, cramps, blurred vision, rash, hair loss, stuffy nose, facial swelling, aggravation of lupus erythematosus, itching, chest pain, back or joint pain, colitis, drug allergy, and liver toxicity.

Ritalin
(Methylphenidate)
Prescribed for attention-deficit hyperactivity disorder, also prescribed for psychological, educational, or social disorders and for narcolepsy and mild depression in the elderly. Methylphenidate is also used in cancer treatment and stroke recovery and for treating hiccups after anesthesia.
Possible side effects: **Most common:** nervousness and inability to sleep. **Least common (rare):** rash, itching, fever, symptoms resembling those of arthritis, appetite loss, nausea, dizziness, abnormal heart rhythm, headache, drowsiness, changes in blood pressure or pulse, chest pain, stomach pain, psychotic reactions, changes in blood components, and loss of some scalp hair.

Zomig
(Triptan-Type Antimigraine Drugs)
Prescribed for migraine. Sumatriptan injection can be used for cluster headaches.

Possible side effects: **Most common:** tightness in the jaw or neck, tingling, a warm or burning sensation, tiredness, dizziness, and fainting. **Least common:** diminished sensitivity to stimulation, heart palpitations, chest pain or pressure, sweating, and muscle aches.

Tussionex Pennkinetic
(Hydrocodone)

Prescribed for cough and other symptoms of a cold or other respiratory condition.

Possible side effects: **Most common:** light-headedness, dizziness, sleepiness, nausea, vomiting, increased sweating, itching, rash, sensitivity to bright light, chills, and dryness of the mouth, nose, or throat. **Least common:** euphoria ("feeling high"), weakness, agitation, uncoordinated muscle movement, disorientation and visual disturbances, minor hallucinations, appetite loss, constipation, facial flushing, rapid heartbeat, palpitations, feeling faint, urinary difficulties, reduced sexual potency, low blood sugar, anemia, yellowing of the skin or whites of the eyes, blurred or double vision, ringing or buzzing in the ears, wheezing, and nasal stuffiness.

Percocet
(Vicodin)

Prescribed for mild to moderate pain.

Possible side effects: **Most common:** light-headedness, dizziness, sleepiness, nausea, vomiting, appetite loss, and increased sweating. **Serious side effects:** Shallow breathing or breathing difficulties.

Appendix IV

FOODS THAT HEAL

-Apples
-Bananas
-Blueberries
-Cantaloupe
-Cranberries
-Grapes
-Grapefruit
-Melons (Honeydew)
-Kiwi
-Lemons/Limes
-Mango
-Nectarines
-Oranges
-Peaches
-Pears
-Pineapple
-Pomegranate
-Prunes
-Raisins
-Strawberries
-Raspberries
-Tangarines
-Watermelon
-Raw Nuts
-Olive Oil
-Almond and Rice Milk
-Organic Skim Milk
-Organic Butter and
 Other Dairy Products
-Whole Grain Foods
 (Whole Wheat Bread)
-Seeds: Flax, Sesame,
 Sunflower, Pumpkin

-Alfalfa
-Artichokes
-Arugula
-Asparagus
-Beets
-Broccoli
-Brussels Sprouts
-Cabbage
-Carrots
-Cauliflower
-Celery
-Cucumber
-Eggplant
-Green Beans
-Kale
-Onions
-Mushrooms
-Parsley
-Parsnips
-Radishes
-Shallots
-Spinach
-Tomato
-Scallions
-Turnips
-Watercress
-Wheatgrass
-Corn
-Potatoes
-Squash
-Lean Skinless Poultry
-Lean Beef, Fish
-Organic Eggs

FOODS TO AVOID

-Sugar
-Salt
-Caffeine
-Alcohol
-White Flour
-White Pasta
-Hydrogenated Oils
-Artificial Sweetners/
 Colors/Preservatives
-Fast Foods
-Refined/Fried Foods
-MSG

DR. JOHNSON'S FAVORITE HEALTH DRESSING

I got this dressing idea from Mr. Paul Bragg. Mr. Bragg was a pioneer in the health food industry and started one of the first health food stores back in the 1930's. For more information, you can go to www.bragg.com.

Ingredients:

Raw organic apple cider vinegar
Extra virgin olive oil
1 packet of Good Seasons Italian dressing mix
Bragg Liquid Aminos

I recommend that you buy the Good Seasons dressing mix with the glass cruet. First, fill the cruet with the raw apple cider vinegar up to the vinegar line. It is very important that you use raw apple cider vinegar and not distilled apple cider vinegar. Raw apple cider vinegar is high in potassium and other minerals that are very beneficial to your body. Next, fill the cruet up to the water line, then add the Good Seasons packet. Fill with the extra virgin olive oil up to the olive oil line, top it off with the Bragg Liquid Aminos, and shake vigorously. This makes an excellent dressing for your salad or coleslaw, and it is one of the most beneficial dressings you can eat.

RECOMMENDED READING

1. <u>SuperFoods Rx</u> by Steven G. Pratt and Kathy Matthews
2. <u>The Maker's Diet</u> by Jordan S. Rubin, Ph.D.
3. <u>Body by God</u> by Ben Lerner
4. <u>Rhinoceros Success</u> by Scott Alexander
5. <u>Body For Life</u> by Bill Philips
6. <u>The Complete Idiot's Guide to Understanding the Brain</u> by Arthur and Mitchell Bard
7. All of Norman Vincent Peale's books

Index

Abdominal exam, 43
Accomodation, 35
Adjustment, 47
Adrenal medulla, 25-27
Advertising, 9
Alcohol, 138
Amygdala, 89
Angular gyrus, 20
Anterior cingulate, 20
Antibiotics, 86
Appleton, 8
Appleton Pharmacy, 9
Arm slap, 39
Arnold-Chiari syndrome, 14
A.S.B.E., 12
Auditory stimulation, 48, 55, 75
AV node, 26, 85

Backstroke, 54
Balance, 56-59
Bariatrics, 14-15
Basal ganglia, 58
Basketball, 3
Benign Paroxysmal Positional Vertigo (BPPV), 57, 58
Biotin, 132
Blepherospasm, 79, 87, 92, 117, 118
Blind spot mapping, 37
Blood pressure, 29, 46

Blood work, 30
Brain, 16, 126, 133
Brainstem, 25- 27, 48, 62-67, 69-109
Broca's speech area, 19, 66
Bruits, 44

Caffeine, 126, 135-137
Calcium, 126-127
Cateacholamides, 25
Calorics, 51
Central integrated state (CIS), 58
Cerebellum, 16, 25, 38, 39, 50, 51, 58-67, 89-109, 112
Chest expansion, 30
Chiropractic neurologist, 10, 25, 55, 70
Chiropractors, 111
Choline, 132
Chromium, 132
Clonazapam (Klonopin), 70, 168
Concentration, 101
Copper, 132-133
Corectasia, 35, 45, 71, 73, 79, 81, 88, 97, 114, 115
Corneal reflex, 34
Cortical spreading depression (CSD), 69
Corneal light reflection, 34-35

Cover/uncover test, 36
Cranial nerve #1, 38
Cranial nerve #3, 35, 36, 121
Cranial nerve #4, 35, 36, 121
Cranial nerve #6, 36, 121
Cranial nerve #7, 38, 121
Cranial nerve #12, 38
CT scan, 86

Davenport, 6, 148-150
Detoxification, 79, 139-140
Diamond Headache Clinic, 79
Diet, 140-141
Dizziness, 51, 56-67, 76
Doppler, 62
Dorsal columns, 113
Drawing, 21

Ear exam, 33
Egocentric vertigo, 57-67
Endolymph, 50, 59, 94
Energy, 86-92
Essential Fatty Acids (EFA),
    127-128
Examination, 28-45
Exophoria, 16, 62-67, 71-81,
    95, 111
Eye exam, 33
Eye exercises, 49, 52

Facial muscles, 38
Fatigue, 82-109
Female brain, 20
Ferris State, 6
Fibromyalgia, 10, 82-109

Folic Acid, 133

Geocentric vertigo, 57-67
Glucose, 31
Gonstead, 6, 11, 12
Grand rounds, 15
Green Bay, WI, 17
Guaifenesin, 108

"happy brain", 20
Heart, 26, 101
Heart exam, 43
Heat, 50, 55
Heel down shin, 41
Heel tap, 41
Heel to toe walk, 41
Hippocampus, 21
HMO, 11, 121

IML, 85
Impulses, 22, 23, 113
Inositol, 133
Insurance companies, 77
Intersegmental traction, 50
Iodine, 133
Irritable bowel syndrome, 101
Iron, 133-134

Journal of the American
    Chiropractic
    Association, 121

Kinocillia, 51, 59
Klonopin, 70, 168

Language, 19
Left brain, 17, 18-27
Letters, 50, 55
Light sensitivity, 25, 69-71, 84
Low back pain, 24

Magnesium, 128-129
"male brain", 20
Manganese, 134
Manipulation, 47, 61-67, 120-124
Manitowoc, 9
Marshfield Clinic, 79
Math, 19
Mayo Clinic, 79
Mazes, 49, 55
Mechanical aptitude, 21
Meclizine, 56-67, 76
Medulla oblongata, 24-25, 68-81
Medical doctors, 10, 14, 111, 120-124
Memory, 21-22
Mesencephalon, 25, 27, 68-109
Metronome, 48
Migraine headache, 1-2, 16-17, 68-81
Mirror imagery, 52, 55
Mozart, 48
Motor strip, 23
MRI, 14, 86
Multiple Sclerosis (MS), 115
Muscle strength, 33
Muscle strength reflexes, 31

NASCAR, 77
Nausea, 60
NCMIC, 123
Network Chiropractic, 12, 13
Neurology, 120
Neurology courses, 15
Neuroplasticity, 23
Neurontin, 114
Newsweek, 22
Niacin, 134
Nicotine, 137
Nociceptive fibers, 27
Non-verbal communication, 20-21
Norepinephrine, 27
Nucleus Tractus Solatarius (NTS), 60
Numbness, 3, 99, 114-115
Nutrition, 125-141

Ocular motion, 36
Olfactory stimulation, 52, 55, 74
Olfactory testing, 38
Optokinetic tape, 36, 60-67, 87-109
Orthopedic exam, 44
Orthopedic surgeon, 10, 111
Oxycodone, 79
Oxygen, 53, 67, 111, 113, 114

Paba, 134
Palmer College, 6, 15
Pathothenic Acid, 135
Paralyzed, 16

Parasthesia, 3, 99, 113
Parietal lobe, 22, 42, 71
Parietal sway, 42-43
Past pointing, 39
Peripheral vision, 36
Pharmacists, 4, 5, 9
Pharmacy, 4
Phosphorus, 135
Physical therapist, 17
Piano, 40
Pinwheel sensation, 32
Pons, 25, 26, 27, 67-109
Posture, 44
Potassium, 135-136
PPO, 11
Prayer, 142-145
"prodome phase", 69
Pronation, 40
Protein, 138
Pulse, 30, 46
Pupil size, 35
Pupillary reflex, 35, 62-67

Rain, 48
Range of motion (ROM), 44
Rapid eye movement, 35
Reading, 21
Rebound headaches, 79
Re-exam, 44-45
Repeat numbers test, 42
Respiration, 29
Right brain, 17, 18-27
Rinne test, 33
Romberg's sign, 38, 61-67, 71-
    81, 91-109, 112

Russian roulette, 70

Salivary PH, 30
SA node, 25-26, 85
Sciatica, 3, 4
Scientists, 22
Selenium, 129
Semicircular canals, 51, 59
Social behavior, 20-21
Somatotopic map, 23
Speech, 19
Spin therapy, 53, 54
Squeeze ball, 54
SpO_2, 29
Stereocillia, 51, 59
Stress, 21
Stroke, 15, 120-124
Supination, 40
Sugar, 137-138
Sweating, 26

Telemarketing, 14
Temporal lobe, 22, 42
T.E.N.S., 50, 75, 112
Thalamus, 74
TMJ, 78
Topomax (topiramate), 70
Treatment, 28, 46-55
Trivial activity, 19
Two point discrimination, 43

Ultimate Eye Filters, 53, 54
Ultrasound, 50
Upper Body Ergometer (UBE),
    52

Urinalysis, 30
Urinate, 27, 83, 121

Vagus nerve, 60-62
V/A ratio, 36, 98
Vertigo, 51, 56-67, 76
Vibratory sensation, 32
Visual imagery, 52, 59, 65
Visual stimulation, 48-50
Vitamin A, 129-130
Vitamin B_1, 130
Vitamin B_2, 130
Vitamin B_6, 130
Vitamin B_{12}, 131
Vitamin C, 131
Vitamin D, 131-132
Vitamin E, 132
Vitamin K, 132

Weber test, 33
Wernicke's area, 19, 66
Wiper blade test, 42

X-ray, 11

Zinc, 129